About the author

Professor Jennie Br[illegible] foremost authorities o[illegible] index and has champio[illegible] ⌐ ιo nutrition for more than twenty-ι ⌐ ⌐ars. Professor of Nutrition at the University of Sydney and past president of the Nutrition Society of Australia, Brand-Miller directs a GI food-labelling program in Australia (www.gisymbol.com. au) with the Juvenile Diabetes Research Foundation to ensure that claims about the GI are scientifically correct and applied only to nutritious foods. Winner of Australia's prestigious ATSE Clunies Ross Award in 2003 for her commitment to advancing science and technology, Brand-Miller is an in-demand speaker, and her laboratory at the University of Sydney is recognised worldwide for cutting-edge research on carbohydrates and health.

Kaye Foster-Powell is an accredited dietitian with more than 20 years' experience in diabetes management. A graduate of the University of Sydney (BSc Master of Nutrition & Dietetics) she has conducted research into the glycemic index of foods and its practical applications. She is a Diabetes Specialist Dietitian with the Nepean Blue Mountains Diabetes Service and co-author the Low GI Diet series.

Doctor Joanna McMillan is a nutritionist-dietitian with a PhD from the University of Sydney; her research looked at the effect of the glycemic index on weight loss. She is now a popular media nutrition spokesperson appearing regularly on TV, radio and in print. Joanna is Director of Dr Joanna (www.drjoanna.com.au), a company specialising in nutrition and healthy living. Having been a fitness instructor for fifteen years, she has helped hundreds of people to change their bodies.

PROFESSOR JENNIE BRAND-MILLER'S

LOWGIDIET
12–week
Weight–loss Plan

**Prof Jennie Brand-Miller • Kaye Foster-Powell
• Dr Joanna McMillan**

hachette
AUSTRALIA

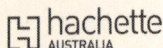

Ⱶ hachette
AUSTRALIA

First published in Australia and New Zealand in 2004
by Hodder Australia
(an imprint of Hachette Australia Pty Limited)
Level 17, 207 Kent Street, Sydney NSW 2000
www.hachette.com.au

Revised editions published in 2006, 2008 and 2011
This updated edition published in 2012

10 9 8 7 6 5 4 3 2 1

National Library of Australia Cataloguing-in-Publication data

Brand Miller, Jennie, 1952-
Low GI diet 12-week weight-loss plan / Jennie Brand-Miller, Kaye Foster-
Powell, Joanna McMillan.
978 0 7336 2671 5 (pbk.)
Previously published: 2008
Includes index.
Reducing diets.
Glycemic index.
Diet therapy.
Food–carbohydrate content.
Dietetics.
Brand Miller, Jennie.
Foster-Powell, Kaye.
McMillan, Joanna.
613.5638

Photography (exercise shots) by Julie Howard
Cover design by Christabella Designs, cover adaptation by Agave Creative
Cover photograph courtesy Getty Images
Back cover portrait © www.gavinjowitt.com
Final text design by Ellie Exarchos; adaptation for this edition by Kirby Jones
Printed in Australia by Griffin Press, Adelaide, an Accredited ISO AS/NZS 4001:2004
Environmental Management Systems printer

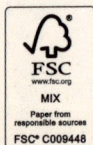

Contents

Introduction

A new approach to dieting

A low-GI diet is a real-life solution to real weight concerns. It delivers long-term weight loss and wellbeing with a healthy eating and exercise program that improves insulin sensitivity and reduces insulin resistance and food cravings. It's the one diet that suits the whole family. It's safe for adults and children, and for people with pre-existing medical conditions such as diabetes, heart disease or PCOS.

In this book, we explain how choosing low-GI carbohydrates—the ones that produce only small fluctuations in your blood glucose and insulin levels—can help you feel fuller for longer and increase your energy levels, making weight loss achievable and sustainable. Lowering your insulin levels is not only a key ingredient in weight loss, but also the secret to long-term health, reducing your risk of heart disease and diabetes. A low-GI diet works for another important reason: it deals not just with your energy intake (what goes in your mouth) but your energy output—energy expenditure and physical activity—getting the legs, not the fingers, to do the walking.

During the '12-week Weight-loss Plan' you will lose at least 250 grams of body fat per week: not water, not muscle, but pure *body fat*, most of it from around the waist. And we promise that you will not be ravenously hungry between meals, you won't be weighing out food and you certainly won't be counting kilojoules. One of the reasons this diet is easy is its unique ability to keep you feeling fuller for longer. It helps control appetite by controlling blood glucose and stimulating the production of the body's own natural appetite suppressants.

This is not a low-carb diet, nor a low-fat diet, nor a high-protein diet: it is flexible and livable and, quite simply, it is a delicious way of eating that incorporates aspects of many ethnic cuisines. It's family friendly too—your partner, your children, younger and older, will be sitting down to the same delicious food as you—only the quantities will vary. And, if you are planning a pregnancy, this is the safest diet for you and your baby right from the time of conception.

How to use this book

The low-GI diet is a lifestyle diet and exercise program aimed at reducing body fat and *keeping it off for life*. Easy to follow and based on making simple substitutions to the way you eat now, it will change the way you eat forever. This book includes:

- The 12-week Weight-loss Plan, based on smart carbs, healthy protein choices and clever moves to help you lose up to 10 per cent of your current body weight

- The tools and tips you need to maintain weight loss for life
- Recipes, meal plans and a menu survival guide for eating out
- Simple practical ways to build more activity into your day
- The GI table, with the GI of your favourite foods.

Chapter 1

Understanding the Low GI Diet

A real-life solution to real weight concerns

If you want to lose body fat and keep it off restrictive dieting isn't the answer. The real goal in losing weight is to shed fat, not muscle mass or body water. And this is what you will achieve with the *Low GI Diet 12-week Weight-loss Plan*.

A new approach that provides a real-life solution, not another temporary fix, is needed to help people achieve sustainable weight loss for life. This is where a low-GI diet is unique. It is the definitive science-based diet that will maximise your muscle mass (increase your engine size), minimise your body fat (decrease the cushioning) and keep you burning the optimal fuel mix (high-octane energy with built-in engine 'protectants') for lifelong weight control. And by optimising your insulin sensitivity and decreasing your insulin levels over the whole day with its combination of healthy eating and exercise, it tackles a key underlying cause that undermines all efforts of weight control.

The 12-week Weight-loss Plan:
- Reduces weight at a faster rate than a low-fat diet
- Decreases body fat, not muscle mass or body water
- Lowers day-long blood glucose and insulin levels
- Increases satiety and minimises hunger pangs
- Maximises the metabolic rate during weight loss
- Reduces the chance of weight regain.

How much weight should you realistically aim to lose?

Setting attainable goals is extremely important. You (and sometimes your doctor) may have completely unrealistic expectations of a weight-loss plan. You might be anticipating excessively rapid weight loss. A well-meaning doctor might encourage you to go back to your 'ideal weight', a body mass index (BMI) between 19 and 25—the so-called 'normal' range. Both of you need to think again and reconsider the rate of weight loss and the absolute amount.

A realistic weight-loss goal that brings about desirable benefits in health and psychological terms is aiming to lose between 5 and 10 per cent of your current weight over a period of 12 weeks so long as you are active. For example, if you currently weigh 100 kilograms, then a weight loss of 5 to 10 kilograms over 12 weeks is realistic, safe and enough to improve your health. If you achieve that and are able to *maintain* that weight loss long term, you are a success!

If you would like to lose more weight, then it is best that you only do that after a period of weight maintenance. Your body needs time to adjust to a lower weight. Each 12-week period of weight loss using this plan (see pages 43–184) should be followed by three to six months of weight maintenance as outlined in 'Doing it for Life' (see pages 185–216), before beginning another 12-week weight-loss period. This alternating strategy takes the pressure off and improves your chances of success. Below you will find our tips for keeping the weight you have lost off. We repeat these tips in the 'Doing it for Life' section . . . but it won't hurt to read it twice.

The Ten Golden Rules of preventing weight regain

1 Don't skip meals (or you will reduce your metabolic rate).
2 Eat a really good breakfast.
3 Eat at least three to four times a day.
4 Limit television to less than 12 hours per week.
5 Choose low-GI carbs at every meal.
6 Eat lean protein sources at every meal.
7 Don't skimp on the fats—just choose healthy ones.
8 Eat seven serves of fruit and vegies every day.
9 Schedule moderate physical activity for 30–60 minutes on six days out of seven.
10 On the seventh day, relax and enjoy.

QUIZ: What is a healthy weight for you?

Women tend to see themselves as being larger than they actually are and aspire to an unattainable size. Men, on the other hand, are better judges of their size but often don't see excess weight as a health problem (real men don't diet!). Assuming you're above a weight at which you feel healthy and comfortable, then it's reasonable to want to change.

Place a tick next to the statements that apply to you.

A My weight (in kilograms) divided by my height squared (in metres) results in a number greater than 25. ☐

B I'm apple-shaped, rather than pear-shaped (i.e. bigger around my waist than I am around my hips). ☐

C Both my parents are overweight. ☐

I have been big most of my life. ☐

D My activity level has declined in the last 5 years. ☐

I think I eat more than I need. ☐

E I suffer from one or more of the following:

elevated blood glucose levels ☐

high blood pressure ☐

blocked arteries ☐

gout ☐

gallstones ☐

sleep apnoea or snoring ☐

osteoarthritis ☐

shortness of breath on exertion ☐

My body weight stops me from doing things I would like to do if I were thinner. ☐

A tick at *A* suggests you are carrying more weight than is normally considered healthy.

What you have calculated here is your body mass index (BMI). It is a measure of your weight in relation to your height. In Caucasian people, a BMI greater than 25 is classified as overweight, and above 30 as obese. Different cut-offs apply for people from other ethnic backgrounds and more muscular people should use a cut-off of 27 as indicating the possibility of being overweight. To calculate your BMI, take your weight (in kilograms) and divide by your height (in metres) squared.

Calculating your BMI

A woman who is 1.5 metres tall and weighs 70 kilograms would calculate her BMI like this

$$\frac{70}{1.5 \times 1.5} = 31$$

A tick at *B* implies an unhealthy distribution of body fat.

It is a large mass of body fat that carries health risks, rather than simply weighing a lot on the scales. A waist measurement greater than 80 centimetres for women and 94 centimetres for men indicates increased health risk due to intra-abdominal fat accumulation. Get the tape measure out and measure your waist circumference—the smallest circumference around your abdomen. This point will be close to your navel but perhaps not exactly on it. Here's what you need to know:

	Overweight and at increased risk of disease	Very overweight and at substantially increased risk of disease
Men	Over 94 cm	Over 102 cm
Women	Over 80 cm	Over 88 cm

Ticks at *C* suggest you may have a genetic predisposition to being overweight.

Scientists recognise people who gain weight much more easily than others, thanks to their genetics as being 'easy gainers'. Weight and body shape are largely the result of genetic background as well as a personal history of dieting and activity (or lack of). So, if you were born with a tendency to be overweight, why does it matter what you eat? Well, genes can be switched on or off. By being choosy about carbohydrates and fats you maximise insulin sensitivity, *up*-regulate the genes involved in burning fat and *down*-regulate those involved in burning carbs. By moving your fuel 'currency exchange' from a 'carbohydrate economy' to a 'fat economy', you increase the opportunity of depleting fat stores over carbohydrate stores. This is exactly what will happen when you begin to eat the foods we suggest in the 12-week Weight-loss Plan.

Ticks at *D* suggest lifestyle factors that may be contributing to your weight.

Energy intake and energy expenditure need to be in balance to maintain a healthy weight. Our current sedentary lifestyles require about 30 to 50 per cent less food energy than the daily demands our parents and grandparents experienced. What changes have caused a reduction in your daily activity? A change of occupation, moving closer to work, giving up smoking (which slows your metabolism), getting a car, an accident that immobilised you? Similarly, can you identify contributors to increasing energy intake such as changed shopping habits, greater wealth, retirement, more reliance on takeaway foods, etc.?

> **'Success breeds success! I love the mental freedom of not having cravings as the best thing of all.' – Diane**
>
> I had never been on a diet or lost a kilo in my life. So, having reached the age of 53, weighing 102 kilos and being pre-diabetic, I decided to adopt a low-GI diet. I read many success stories, but never did I think I would be as successful as these people. I couldn't imagine myself as losing weight and being lighter; I couldn't really remember weighing less.
>
> Well, only 12 weeks later, I weigh less than 90 kilos! I stare at the scales every morning in amazement. It has become an incentive to continue, as success breeds success! I never imagined I would be able to cut down my chocolate habit to next to nothing, but it has been so easy.

Ticks at _E_ suggest that your weight is affecting your health and daily life.

It isn't true that to reach and maintain optimal health and personal happiness you have to be thin. Health and vitality come in all shapes and sizes. It is that deep, central body fat that seems to be linked with disease. The good news is that when an overweight person loses just 5 to 10 per cent of their body weight and keeps it off, many of the adverse medical consequences of being overweight subside.

How a low-GI diet helps you lose weight

As we explain in more detail on page 13, eating low-GI foods, the basis for the low-GI diet, has two important advantages for people trying to lose weight:

- These smart carb foods help you overcome hunger because they fill you up and keep you satisfied for longer than their high-GI counterparts.
- They reduce insulin levels and help you burn more body fat and less muscle, so your metabolic rate is higher.

A low-GI diet helps you overcome hunger

A low-GI diet is based on an important scientifically proven fact—that carb foods with low GI values are more filling than their high-GI counterparts. They not only give you a greater feeling of fullness instantly, but delay hunger pangs for longer and reduce food intake during the remainder of the day. In contrast, foods with a high GI can actually stimulate appetite sooner, increasing consumption at the next meal. Because low-GI foods have a slow rate of digestion and absorption, foods reach lower parts of the small intestine, stimulating the secretion of powerful 'satiety factors' that help people feel satisfied. A low-GI diet also harnesses nature's own appetite suppressants so that weight loss is easier to achieve than ever before.

A low-GI diet reduces insulin levels and thus helps you burn more body fat and less muscle

You are probably familiar with the hormone insulin. It is the one that is missing in people with type 1 diabetes and needs to be injected daily for survival. Most of us have the opposite problem—we have far too much of it circulating at any one time. This is especially true of overweight people, those with type 2 diabetes or family history of it, and indeed any man or woman with a 'beer gut' or 'pot belly'.

Excess fat around the waist causes a form of inertia or resistance to insulin's action, resulting in the need to secrete more and more insulin to overcome the hurdle (a bit like shouting to make a deaf person hear). These high circulating levels of insulin spell trouble called 'insulin resistance' (also known as the metabolic syndrome or Syndrome X). By losing weight, you can substantially reduce your insulin levels, especially if you choose low-GI carbs in place of your usual carbohydrate sources.

Having persistently high insulin levels is likely to make you fatter and fatter, undermining all your efforts at weight control.

Having persistently high insulin levels is likely to make you fatter and fatter, undermining all your efforts at weight control. It is the very reason why people with diabetes find it so hard to lose weight. The higher your insulin levels, the more carbohydrate you burn at the expense of fat.

Why insulin resistance is a big deal

If your doctor has told you that you have high blood pressure and 'a touch of sugar' (pre-diabetes or impaired glucose tolerance) then you probably have the insulin resistance syndrome. The higher your insulin levels, the more carbohydrate you burn at the expense of fat. This is because insulin has two powerful actions: one is to 'open the gates' so that glucose can flood into the cells and be used as the source of energy. The second role of insulin is to *inhibit* the release of fat from fat stores. Furthermore, the burning of glucose inhibits the burning of fat and vice versa.

These actions persist even in the face of insulin resistance because the body overcomes the extra hurdle by just pumping out more insulin into the blood. Unfortunately, the level that finally drives glucose into the cells is two to ten times more than is needed to switch off the use of fat as a source of fuel. If insulin is high all day long, as it is in insulin resistant and overweight people, then the cells are constantly forced to use glucose as their fuel source, drawing it from either the blood or stored glycogen. Blood glucose therefore swings from low to high and back again, playing havoc with our appetite and triggering the release of stress hormones. Our meagre stores of carbohydrate in the liver and muscles also undergo major fluctuations over the course of the day. When you don't get much chance to use fat as a source of fuel, it is not surprising that fat stores accumulate wherever they can:

- Inside the muscle cells (a sign of insulin resistance)
- In the blood (this is called high triglycerides or TG and is often seen in people with diabetes or the metabolic syndrome)
- In the liver (non-alcoholic fatty liver, NAFL), and
- Around the waist (the proverbial pot belly).

The real deal on carbohydrates and the GI

Carbohydrate is a vital source of energy found in all plants and foods that come from plants, such as fruit, vegetables, cereals and grains. The simplest form of carbohydrate is glucose, which is:

- A universal fuel for our body cells
- The only fuel source for our brain, red blood cells and a growing foetus, and
- The main source of energy for our muscles during strenuous exercise.

Our bodies rev on carbs. When you eat bread, fruit and grain foods such as rice or pasta, your body converts them into a sugar called glucose during digestion. It is this glucose that is absorbed from your intestine and becomes the fuel that circulates in your bloodstream. As the level of blood glucose rises after you have eaten a meal, your pancreas gets the message to release a powerful hormone called insulin. Insulin drives glucose out of the blood and into the cells. Once inside, glucose will be channelled into various pathways simultaneously—it will be used as an immediate source of energy, or converted to glycogen (a storage form of glucose), or converted into fat. Insulin also turns off the use of fat as the cell's energy source. For this reason, lowering insulin levels is one of the secrets to life-long health. However, cutting carbs out altogether is *not* the answer.

What we know today is that not all carbs are created equal. In fact, they can behave quite differently in our

The glycemic index is today's dietary power tool.

bodies. The glycemic index or GI is how we describe this difference, ranking carbs (sugars and starches) according to their effect on blood glucose levels. After testing hundreds of foods around the world, scientists have now found that foods with a low GI will have less of an effect on blood glucose levels than foods with a high GI. High-GI foods tend to cause spikes in glucose levels whereas low-GI foods tend to cause gentle rises.

The key to understanding GI is the rate of digestion

Foods containing carbohydrates that break down quickly during digestion have the highest GI values. The blood glucose response is fast and high. In other words, the glucose (or sugar) in the bloodstream increases rapidly. Conversely, foods that contain carbohydrates that break down slowly, releasing glucose gradually into the bloodstream, have a low GI value. An analogy we like to use is the popular fable of the tortoise and the hare. The hare, just like high-GI foods, speeds away but loses the race to the tortoise with his slow and steady pace. Similarly, the slow and steady low-GI foods produce a smooth blood glucose curve without wild fluctuations. For most people, the foods with low GI values have advantages over those with high GI values. However, in elite sport, there are times when a high-GI carbohydrate will be the best choice.

Switching to eating mainly low-GI carbs that slowly trickle glucose into your blood stream keeps your energy levels perfectly balanced and means you will feel fuller for longer between meals. The whole idea is to replace highly refined carbohydrate such as white bread, sugary sweets and rice bubbles with less processed carbs such as grainy bread, pasta, beans, fruit and vegetables.

Why low-GI smart carbs help you lose weight

Our own weight loss studies at the University of Sydney, as well as research from Harvard University and Hotel Dieu Hospital, Paris, France confirm that the GI helps people lose weight, specifically that dangerous fat around the belly we mentioned earlier. There is concrete evidence that a low-GI diet increases the rate of weight loss compared to a conventional low-fat diet. What's more, the fat loss is maintained long term. That is a critically important point because it is where the other diets fail. Let's take a close look at all the facts supporting our healthy low-GI diet.

1 Overcoming hunger

The low-GI diet is based on an important scientifically proven fact that foods with low GI values will keep you feeling fuller for longer than their high-GI counterparts. They not only give you a greater feeling of fullness instantly, but delay hunger pangs for longer and reduce food intake during the remainder of the day. In contrast, foods with a high GI can actually stimulate appetite sooner, increasing consumption at the next meal.

There are several explanations: low-GI foods remain longer in the gut and reach much lower parts of the small intestine, triggering receptors that produce natural appetite suppressants. Many of these receptors are present only in the lower gut. It doesn't take a genius to appreciate that a food that empties rapidly from the stomach and gets digested and absorbed in minutes won't satisfy for hours on end.

2 Fat loss is faster with low-GI foods

There are now a dozen or more studies showing that people who eat low-GI foods lose more body fat than those eating high-GI foods. In one study conducted by Harvard scientists, overweight adults were instructed to follow either a conventional high-fibre, low-fat diet or a low-GI diet containing more good fats and low-GI carbs. The low-GI group's diet emphasised foods such as porridge, eggs, low-fat dairy produce and pasta. In contrast, the low-fat diet emphasised high-fibre cereal products, potatoes and rice. Both diets contained the same number of kilojoules and were followed for 18 months (6 months of intense intervention and 12 months of follow-up). At the end changes in weight were similar in both groups. But, among the people who had high insulin levels (half of them), those on a low-GI diet lost nearly 6 kilograms of weight compared to only 1 kilogram on the conventional low-fat diet. Moreover, they lost three times more body fat and had greater improvements in cardiovascular risk factors.

In our own research unit at the University of Sydney, we have made similar findings in a group of young overweight adults who followed one of the four popular diets. To ensure dietary compliance, we gave them most of the food they needed for the whole 12-week period. At the end, we found that weight and body fat loss were over 50 per cent greater in those following our low-GI diet than those following the conventional low-fat approach. Those instructed to follow a high-protein diet also lost more body fat but showed adverse effects on blood lipids. Fortunately, the cholesterol-raising effect of the high-protein diet could be prevented by simultaneous consumption of low-GI carbs.

Why do low-GI diets work so well for weight loss? The most important reason is likely to be the effect on day-long insulin levels—low-GI foods result in lower levels of insulin over the course of the whole day.

The hormone insulin is not only involved in regulating blood glucose levels, but also plays a key part in fat storage. High levels of insulin mean the body is forced to burn carbohydrate rather than fat. Thus, over the day, even if the total energy burnt is the same, the proportions of fat to carbohydrate are different. Oxidising carbohydrate won't really help you lose weight, but burning fat will.

These are not idle claims. Dr Emma Stevenson's research with Loughborough University in the UK demonstrated over and over that, compared with healthy conventional meals, low-GI meals were associated with greater fat oxidation during episodes of gentle exercise in overweight volunteers.

The 'famine reaction'

The invisible enemy of any dieting effort is a natural physiological phenomenon that makes it progressively more difficult for dieters to keep losing weight, and even more difficult for them to keep it off. Dr Amanda Sainsbury-Salis, obesity researcher at the Garvan Institute in Sydney, calls this the 'famine reaction': it's a survival mechanism that's been helping the human race to survive famines and food shortages for millions of years. The famine reaction is the reason why after each dieting effort, you end up doing battle with ravenous hunger, craving for fattening foods, guilt-ridden binge-eating, lethargy, weight plateauing and rapid rebound weight gain. These are all classic signs of the famine reaction in full swing. It has nothing to do with lack of commitment or willpower. It's why conventional dieting advice fails.

In her book *The Don't Go Hungry Diet*, Dr Sainsbury-Salis explains the origin of these telltale symptoms—a naturally occurring hormone called neuropeptide Y. Its secretion causes irrepressible increases in hunger, the hallmark feature of the famine reaction, but also acts to prevent further weight loss and promote fat accumulation, regardless of whether or not the person continues to follow a program of diet and physical activity. Neuropeptide Y is just one of a whole army of hormones and brain chemicals that bring on the famine reaction. All conspire to make sure you hit the wall of resistance to further weight loss. Drinking water, moving more and eating more fibre only serve to make the famine reaction stronger: more hunger, more cravings, more lethargy, an even slower metabolic rate and longer plateau.

How do you switch off the famine reaction? Simple. It can be switched off by *eating freely*, eating to appetite, eating as much as you want. In other words, eating enough to satisfy your physical hunger, including your favourite foods. Nothing more complicated than that. The science behind this concept is brand new but rock solid. And it provides another explanation for the long-term success of our low-GI diet, i.e., a diet underpinned by *eating to appetite*, enjoying foods that make you feel fuller for longer, because they take many more hours to be digested and absorbed.

The 'fat brake'

Here is another crucial piece of scientific research with the potential to change your life for the better. According to Dr Amanda Sainsbury-Salis, not only does your body have the potential to mount a famine reaction to stop you losing weight, it also possesses a remarkable system that protects you from gaining weight. She calls it the 'fat brake'. If you can pick up the fat brake signals, it will actually be difficult for you to get fat. Just as there are brain chemicals and hormones that control the famine reaction, there is an opposing army of brain chemicals controlling the fat brake. The commander is a hormone called leptin that has the opposite effects to neuropeptide Y. It acts to blunt the appetite, increase the tendency to be active and boost the metabolic rate. So not only should you heed signals that say 'eat more' but also those that say 'eat less' and 'don't eat yet'.

People who are overweight have been shown to have high glycogen (carbohydrate) stores that undergo major fluctuations during the day. This suggests that glycogen is a more important source of fuel for them. If glycogen is being depleted and replenished on a regular basis (before and after each meal, for example), it is displacing fat from the engine. Each meal restores glycogen (especially if the food has a high GI value) and the cycle repeats itself. Carbohydrate 'balance', as it's called, is turning out to be one of the best predictors of future weight gain.

The benefits of a low-GI diet for weight control go beyond appetite and fat burning. When you first begin a diet, your metabolic rate drops in response to the reduction in food intake, which makes weight loss slower and slower. Research shows your metabolic rate drops much less, however, on a low-GI diet than a conventional diet. If your engine revs are higher, you'll not only lose weight faster, you'll also be much less likely to regain it.

The fall in metabolic rate that occurs whenever we restrict our energy intake is part of our body's natural response to food scarcity. This brings us to two new and profound concepts in the obesity research field, described in lay terms as the 'famine reaction' and the 'fat brake'.

There are even more good reasons to choose a low-GI diet for weight loss:

- When you first begin a diet, your metabolic rate drops in response to the reduction in food intake, which makes weight loss hard to sustain. Your metabolic rate drops much less, however, on the low-GI diet than a conventional low-fat diet. So your engine revs are higher.

- A low-GI diet brings about a reduction in the dangerous fat—around the abdomen—with minimal loss of muscle.
- Large-scale studies in people with diabetes have found that diets including low-GI carbs are linked not only to lower waist circumference, but also to better diabetes control.

Protein, health and a low-GI diet

Protein is an important part of a low-GI diet because it makes us feel more satisfied immediately after eating and reduces hunger between meals. You'll find that you will be eating all the protein you need or feel like eating on the 12-week Weight-loss Plan. We recommend lean meat, fish, chicken as well as eggs and low-fat dairy foods in our menus. But you don't have to eat meat, chicken or fish to get enough protein. Plant proteins can provide you with all the essential and non-essential amino acids you need so long as you eat a wide variety of foods and make sure that you include plenty of legumes (pulses), foods rich in soy protein such as tofu, plus nuts and seeds, wholegrains and vegetables in your diet. If you eat dairy foods and eggs as well, it's even easier.

The other side of the energy equation

If you don't build physical activity into your life, you have very little chance of changing your body shape for life. You can certainly lose weight through dieting alone, but

The people most likely to keep the weight off are those who make exercise a natural part of life.

chances are you will regain any weight lost (and probably gain more) over the weeks and months after you stop actively 'dieting'.

Exercising while you lose weight will help you to maximise fat loss and minimise lean muscle loss. This means you get *leaner faster*. Since you maintain or even build muscle you can help to prevent the drop in your metabolic rate caused by your decreasing body weight. This, in turn, means that you burn more energy each and every minute of every day. All good news!

But the benefits don't stop there. Fit people *burn more fat*. So once you have lost weight, continuing to exercise makes your body a fat-burning machine which is much more effective at resisting weight regain. Furthermore, exercise and the amount of muscle you have affects your body's ability to respond to insulin—fit people need less insulin to do the job of maintaining blood glucose levels because their muscles are primed and trained to respond quickly and effectively to incoming fuel. Alongside a healthy low-GI diet, these changes maximise your chances of maintaining a lean, fit body for life.

A low-GI diet plus physical activity maximises your chances of maintaining a lean, fit body for life.

Chapter 2

The Seven Guidelines of the Low GI Diet

CHOOSING LOW-GI FOODS IS ONE OF THE MOST IMPORTANT dietary choices you can make. As well as identifying your best low-GI smart carb choices, our seven dietary guidelines below give you a blueprint for eating for life.

1 Eat seven or more servings of fruit and vegetables every day.

2 Eat low-GI breads and cereals.

3 Eat legumes, including soybeans, chickpeas and lentils, more often.

4 Eat nuts more regularly.

5 Eat more fish and seafood.

6 Eat lean red meats, poultry and eggs.

7 Eat low-fat dairy products.

Low GI: 55 or less
Moderate or medium GI: 56–69
High GI: 70 or more

1 Eat seven or more servings of fruit and vegetables every day

Why?

Being high in fibre and therefore filling, and low in fat (apart from olives and avocado, which contain some 'good' fats), fruit and vegetables play a central role in a low-GI diet. In addition to protecting you against diseases (ranging from high blood pressure through to cancer), they are bursting with nutrients that will give you a glow of good health, such as:

- Beta-carotene—the plant precursor of vitamin A, used to maintain healthy skin and eyes. A diet rich in beta-carotene may even lessen skin damage caused by UV rays. Apricots, peaches, mangoes, carrots, broccoli and sweet potato are particularly rich in beta-carotene.

- Vitamin C—nature's water soluble anti-oxidant. Anti-oxidants are a bit like your personal bodyguard, protecting your body cells from the damage that can be caused by pollutants in our environment and which also occurs as a natural part of ageing. Guava, capsicum, orange, kiwi fruit and rockmelon are especially rich in vitamin C.

- Anthocyanins—the purple and red pigments in blueberries, capsicum, beetroot and eggplant which also function as antioxidants, minimising the damage to cell membranes that occurs with ageing.

How much?

Aim to eat at least two serves of fruit and five serves of vegetables every day, preferably of three or more different colours. A serve is about one medium-sized piece of fruit, half a cup of cooked vegies or one cup raw.

Which vegetables are lower GI?

Most vegetables contain so little carbohydrate that they don't have a GI value. Potato is a notable exception, however—generally it has a high GI. There are some low-GI varieties like the Carisma potato with a GI of 55, peeled and boiled. If you are a big potato eater, try to replace some of the potato in your diet with these lower GI alternatives.

Sweetcorn (GI 46–48)

Sweetcorn contains folic acid, potassium, the anti-oxidant vitamins A and C, and dietary fibre. Add canned or frozen kernels to soups, stews, relishes, salsas and salads, or simply enjoy it on the cob. For the best flavour, buy fresh corn with the husk intact, because the sugar in the kernels transforms into starch the moment the husk is removed.

Corn is often used as a base for gluten-free products. However, many products manufactured from corn such as cornflakes, cornmeal and corn pasta do not have a low GI. Check the GI tables first (see pages 271–316).

Sweet potato (orange-fleshed) (GI 61)

Sweet potatoes are an excellent source of beta-carotene, vitamin C and dietary fibre. They make a great substitute for potatoes. Peel them or simply scrub the skins and steam, boil, bake or microwave. Try mashing them with a little mustard seed oil or wrapping them in foil and cooking on the barbecue. They also make a tasty addition to casseroles, stir-fries and soups and (roasted first) to salads.

Taro (GI 54)

Taro is a traditional slowly digested food eaten widely throughout the Pacific Islands. It has a dry texture, a flavour similar to sweet potato and can be used the same way. Before cooking, peel off the thick skin wearing rubber gloves (as the juice has been known to cause skin irritation), then cut into wedges and steam, boil or bake.

Yam (GI 37)

Yam, with its thick brownish skin and creamy flesh, is high in fibre and nutrient dense. It's a good source of vitamin C and potassium. Similar to sweet potato and taro but with an earthier flavour, yam can be steamed, microwaved, boiled or baked in wedges or roasted and added to salads.

Which fruits are low GI?

Most fruits have a low GI thanks to the presence of the low-GI sugar fructose, soluble and insoluble fibres and acids (which may slow down stomach emptying).

The lowest GI fruits—apples, pears, all citrus (oranges, grapefruit, mandarins) and stone fruits (peaches, nectarines, plums, apricots)—are those grown in temperate climates. Generally, the more acidic a fruit the lower the GI. Tropical fruits such as pineapple, paw paw, rockmelon and watermelon tend to have intermediate GI values but they are excellent sources of anti-oxidants and in average servings their glycemic load is low.

Most berries have so little carbohydrate that their GI is impossible to test. Strawberries have been tested, however, and they are low GI. Enjoy them by the bowl.

2 Eat low-GI breads and cereals

Why?

What affects the GI of your diet the most? The type of bread and cereals you eat. Mixed grain breads, sourdough, traditional rolled oats, cracked wheat, pearl barley, pasta, noodles and certain types of rice are just some examples of low-GI cereal foods. The slow digestion and absorption of these foods will fill you up more, trickle fuel into your engine at a more useable rate and keep you satisfied for longer.

How much?

Most people need at least five serves of grains each day (very active people need much more), where a serve is one slice of bread, 30 grams of dry cereal, or one-third of a cup of rice or small grains such as bulgur.

Bread

If bread forms a large part of your diet, one of the most important changes you can make to lower the GI of your diet is to choose a low-GI bread. Choose a really grainy bread, granary bread, stoneground wholemeal bread, sourdough bread, or bread made from chickpea or other legume-based flours. Small, specialty bakers are the most likely places you will find them. Some healthy low-GI choices are listed below and you'll find more in the tables at the back of the book.

Grainy breads—Grainy breads contain *lots* of 'grainy bits', tend to be chewy and are nutritionally superior, containing high levels of fibre, vitamins, minerals and phytoestrogens.

Choose breads made with whole cereal grains such as barley, rye, triticale (a wheat and rye hybrid), oats, soy and cracked wheat, and have seeds such as sunflower seeds and linseeds added.

Pumpernickel—Also known as rye kernel bread, pumpernickel contains 80–90 per cent whole and cracked rye kernels. It is dense and compact and is usually sold thinly sliced. The main reason for its low GI value is its content of whole cereal grains.

Sourdough—Sourdough results from the deliberately slow fermentation of flour by yeasts which produces a build-up of organic acids.

These acids give sourdough its characteristic taste. This flavourful low-GI bread is a popular choice for sandwiches (its compact structure keeps the sandwich intact), makes great toast and is generally considered acceptable by those family members who absolutely insist on white bread. The flavour blends well with all kinds of fillings and toppings, making it ideal for lunch boxes, snacks and to serve with soups, salads and main meals.

Stoneground wholemeal or whole-wheat breads—This means that the flour has been milled from the entire wheat berry (the germ, endosperm and the bran) and that the milling process uses a method of slowly grinding the grain with a burrstone instead of high-speed metal rollers to distribute the germ oil more evenly. Virtually none of the ingredients packaged in the wheat berry get lost in this processing method and that is why this bread is such a rich source of several B vitamins, iron, zinc and dietary fibre.

Fruit loaf—The GI of fruit loaf is relatively low because of the part substitution of wheat flour (high GI) with dried fruits (lower GI). The presence of sugar in the dough also limits gelatinisation of the starch.

Chapatti-baisen—Chapatti is unleavened or slightly leavened bread that looks rather like pita bread. It is widely eaten throughout the Indian subcontinent and is available in Indian restaurants worldwide. While it is often made with wheat flour, it is also made from baisen or chickpea flour, giving it a significantly lower GI than when made from wheat flour, due to the nature of the starch. All legumes, including chickpeas, have a higher proportion of amylose starch than that found in cereal grains. So, before you order, ask what flour was used.

Breakfast cereals

Traditional rolled oats cooked into porridge is about the closest most of us come to a true grainy cereal. Although many commercial cereals are labelled 'grainy', the processing they have undergone has destroyed the original physical form of the grain. Some commercial breakfast cereals, however, still do have a low GI thanks to a less extreme degree of processing and the presence of other factors (such as protein or soluble fibre) which slow down digestion. Or try making your own muesli using rolled oats and a mixture of dried fruit, nuts and seeds.

Wholegrain and low GI are not the same

When it comes to what manufacturers put on the label, there's no international definition of 'wholegrain'. Food Standards Australia and New Zealand (FSANZ) have expanded the legal definition for packaging labels to allow foods in which the intact grain or the dehulled, ground, milled, cracked or flaked grain, where the constituents—endosperm, germ and bran—'are present in such proportions that represent the typical ratio of those fractions occurring in the whole cereal' to be labelled wholegrain. Unfortunately, many of the processes increase the GI of the cereal, so, if there's no GI rating on the label, follow our rule of thumb: if you can't see the grains, don't assume it's low GI.

Other low-GI cereal grains

Barley (pearl barley GI 25)

One of the oldest cultivated cereals, barley is very nutritious and high in soluble fibre, which helps to reduce the post-meal rise in blood glucose and lowers its GI. Look for products such as pearl barley to use in soups, stews and pilafs, and barley flakes or rolled barley, which have a light, nutty flavour and can be cooked as a cereal and used in baked goods and stuffing.

Bulgur (GI 48)

Also known as cracked wheat, bulgur is made from wheat grains that have been hulled and steamed before grinding to crack the grain. The whole-wheat grain in bulgur remains virtually intact—it is simply cracked—and the wheat germ and bran are retained, which preserves nutrients and lowers the GI. Bulgur is used as the base of the Middle Eastern salad tabbouli, but can also be used in pilafs, vegie burgers, stuffing, stews, salads and soups or as a cereal.

Noodles

Many Asian noodles such as Hokkien, udon and rice vermicelli have low to intermediate GI values because of their dense texture, whether they are made from wheat or rice flour. Lungkow bean thread noodles, also called cellophane noodles or green bean vermicelli, are a smart carb choice. These shiny fine white noodles are usually sold in bundles wrapped in cellophane in the Asian food aisle of your supermarket or in an Asian food market. Soak them in hot water for 10 minutes then add to stir-fries and salads as they tend to absorb the flavours of other foods they are cooked with. The reason for their low GI includes their legume origin (they are made from mung beans) and their noodle shape and dense texture.

Oats (Rolled oats GI 59)

Rolled oats are grainy oats that have been hulled, steamed and flattened; this popular cereal grain lowers the GI of oatmeal, muesli, biscuits, bread and meatloaf. Oat bran also has a low GI.

Pasta

Pastas of any shape or size have a fairly low GI and are a great stand-by for quick meals. Served with vegetables or tomato sauce and/or accompaniments such as olive oil, fish and lean meat, plenty of vegetables and small amounts of cheese, a pasta meal gives you a healthy balance of carbs, fats and proteins. Pasta should be slightly firm (al dente) and offer some resistance when you are chewing it. Not only does it taste better this way but it has a lower GI as overcooking boosts the GI.

Most pasta is made from semolina (finely cracked wheat) which is milled from very hard wheat (durum) with a high protein content. There is some evidence that thicker types of pasta have a lower GI than thinner types because of the dense consistency and perhaps because they cook more slowly and are less likely to be overcooked. Adding egg to fresh pasta lowers the GI by increasing the protein content.

Note: Canned spaghetti has a higher GI value.

Rice

Rice can have a high GI value (80–109) or a low GI value (50–55) depending on the variety and, in particular, its amylose content.

Basmati, Doongara CleverRice and Moolgiri medium grain rice contain higher proportions of amylose (a type of starch that we digest more slowly), which produces a lower glycemic response, is more compact in structure and more slowly digested.

Waxy or glutinous rice, often used for rice desserts as it becomes sticky when cooked, has a high GI. Arborio rice, which is especially good for making Italian risotto, releases its starch during cooking and has a high GI as a result. Eat less of these kinds of rice.

Sushi—These bite-size parcels of raw or smoked fish, chicken, tofu and/or pickled, raw or cooked vegetables wrapped in seaweed with rice that has been seasoned with vinegar, salt and sugar, make ideal snacks and light meals. Even though the rice used to make sushi in Australia and New Zealand is short grain and somewhat sticky, sushi still has a low GI value. In addition, sushi made with salmon and tuna boosts your intake of the healthy omega-3 fats.

'This is such the right way to go! I am a completely different person now.' – Adriana

I have tried everything in the past—you mention it and I have done it: from high-protein regimens to eating pineapple and tuna every day or simply starving. I did not understand what was happening in my body and what was making me eat so much of the wrong types of food. The low-glycemic concept came to me around two years ago and since then my life changed completely. I have forgotten what it is like to be in the yo-yo cycle, what it is like to crave food, being moody or having regular headaches when I am hungry. I now have excellent control of what I eat and I am a healthy weight. There are two reasons for this: I am no longer addicted to the high-GI carbohydrates and I do not have to rely on my will to make this one work. This is the best way to start a healthy lifestyle, achieve a healthy weight, keep it forever and prevent many chronic diseases proven to be related to overweight and obesity. Eating mostly low GI and doing regular exercise was the way to go for me. Give yourself a chance to experience this amazing way of living!

Rye (GI 34)
Whole kernel rye is used to make certain breads, including pumpernickel and some crispbreads. Rye flakes can be used in a similar way to rolled oats: you can eat them as a cooked cereal or sprinkle them over bread before you bake it.

Whole-wheat kernels (GI 41)
Wheat provides a staple food to half the world's population. Soak wholewheat overnight and simmer for about an hour to use as a base for pilaf. Some people enjoy wheat bran as a cooked breakfast cereal. Cream of wheat is made from very fine semolina; you can use it as a breakfast cereal or in puddings, custards, soufflés and soups.

3 Eat legumes including soybeans, chickpeas and lentils more often

Why?
You need to look no further than legumes for a low-GI food that is easy on the budget, versatile, filling, nutritious and low in kilojoules. Legumes are high in fibre, too—both soluble and insoluble—and are packed with nutrients, providing a valuable source of protein, carbohydrate, B vitamins, folate, iron, zinc and magnesium. Whether you buy dried beans, lentils and chickpeas and cook them yourself at home, or opt for the very convenient, time-saving canned varieties, you are choosing one of nature's lowest GI foods.

Legumes have two particularly special properties among their armour of health benefits. The first is their content of phytochemicals—natural plant chemicals that possess antiviral, antifungal, antibacterial and anti-cancer properties. Plus, legumes are prebiotics. This means that they provide food for our gut bacteria or 'intestinal flora', keeping our digestive system healthy.

Try using beans in place of grains or potatoes. You could try serving a bean salsa with fish or cannellini bean purée with grilled meat. Butter beans can also make a delicious potato substitute. Although they will keep indefinitely, it is best to use dried legumes within one year of purchase.

How much?

At least twice a week as a main meal such as bean soup, chickpea curry or lentil patties, or as a light meal such as beans on toast, mixed bean salad, or pea and ham soup.

Beans

When you add beans to meals and snacks, you reduce the overall GI of your diet and gain important health benefits. Beans are available dried or in cans. Young beans cook

Baked beans—GI 49

Black-eyed beans—GI 42

Butter beans—GI 31

Cannellini beans—GI 31

Haricot beans—GI 33

Lima beans—GI 32

Mung beans—GI 39

Red kidney beans—GI 36

faster than old ones and will also be more vividly coloured. Substitute one 400-gram can of beans for three-quarters of a cup of dried beans. Dried beans usually have a lower GI than canned, but using cans is infinitely more convenient and the GI remains low.

Chickpeas (GI 28)

These large, caramel-coloured legumes are popular in Middle Eastern and Mediterranean dishes. You can buy them in cans or as dried beans. To cook chickpeas, first place them in a bowl, cover them with plenty of cold water and soak them overnight. Drain the water, then put the chickpeas in a saucepan and cover them with clean water. Bring the beans to the boil for 10 minutes then simmer for 1½ hours until they're tender to bite.

You can also roast and salt whole chickpeas for a delicious snack food. Ground chickpea flour (also called gram flour or baisen) is used to make unleavened Indian bread.

Lentils (GI 26)

Lentils are rich in protein, fibre and B vitamins. All colours and types have a similar low GI value, which is increased slightly if you opt to buy them canned and add them at the end of cooking time. Lentils are one food that people with diabetes should learn to love—they can eat them until the cows come home. In fact we have found that no matter how much of them people eat they have only a small effect on blood glucose levels. Lentils have a fairly bland, earthy flavour and are best prepared with onions, garlic and spices. Use them as a 'bed' for grilled fish or meat. They are great for thickening any kind of soup or extending meat casseroles.

Channa dhal (also called Bengal gram dhal) are husked, split, polished Bengal gram, the most common type of gram lentil in India. They are often cooked with a pinch of asafoetida (an Indian spice) to make them easier to digest.

Soybeans (GI 14)

Soybeans and soy products have been a staple part of Asian diets for thousands of years and are an excellent source of protein. They are also rich in fibre, iron, zinc and vitamin B. They are lower in carbohydrate and higher in fat than other legumes but the majority of the fat is polyunsaturated. Soy is also a rich source of phytochemicals, phytoestrogens in particular, which are plant oestrogens with a structure similar to the female hormone oestrogen. Some studies link phytoestrogens with improvements in blood cholesterol levels, relief from menopausal symptoms and lower rates of cancer.

Split peas (GI 32)

Split peas are prepared from a variety of the common garden pea with the husk removed. They may be yellow or green. They take about an hour to cook after soaking and are traditionally used in pea and ham soups or for making an Indian dhal.

> ### 'I couldn't believe that I was losing weight by eating.' – Karen
>
> I would like to say thank you to the whole GI team. I have been a yo-yo dieter for 20 years and have gradually gained more and more weight. I began to do a 'no no', that is not eat, thinking that this would help me to lose weight. This only led to pre-diabetes and gaining much, much more weight. I tried every diet and exercise regime, only to keep gaining weight. It wasn't until I began to get low blood glucose levels and often felt like I was going to pass out that I saw my doctor. But he didn't help, he just said to 'keep dieting'. So I persisted for the sake of my hubby and my children—42 is too young to be on the road to diabetes and heart disease. My family need their wife and mum. Then I had had enough and went to a different GP who told me about the GI team and the low-GI diet. I was amazed to discover that within a week of beginning the diet (plus some gentle exercise), I began shedding the kilos. Moreover, my blood glucose levels were normalising finally after ten years.

4   Eat nuts more regularly

Why?

Although nuts are high in fat, it is mainly polyunsaturated and monounsaturated so they make a healthy substitute for less nutritious high saturated-fat snacks such as potato chips, chocolate and cookies.

Nuts are one of the richest sources of vitamin E, which, with the selenium they contain, works as an anti-oxidant. Selenium helps guard against harmful UV rays to reduce damage caused by the sun and premature ageing of your skin.

How much?

Aim for a small handful of nuts (30 grams) most days.

Here are some easy ways to eat more nuts:

- Use nuts and seeds in food preparation. For example, use toasted cashews or sesame seeds in a chicken stir-fry; sprinkle walnuts or pine nuts over a salad; top fruity desserts or granola with almonds.
- Use hazelnut spread on bread or try peanut, almond or cashew butter rather than butter or margarine.
- Sprinkle a mixture of ground nuts and linseeds over cereal or salads, or add to baked goods such as muffins.

5 Eat more fish and seafood

Why?

Fish does not have a GI as it is a source of protein, not carbohydrate. Increased fish consumption is linked to a reduced risk of coronary heart disease, improvements in mood, lower rates of depression, better blood fat levels and enhanced immunity. Just one serving of fish a week may reduce the risk of a fatal heart attack by 40 per cent. The likely protective components of fish are the very long chain omega-3 fatty acids. Our bodies only make small amounts of these fatty acids and so we rely on dietary sources, especially fish and seafood, for them.

How much?

One to three meals of fish each week.

Which fish is best?

- Oily fish, which tend to have darker-coloured flesh and a stronger flavour, are the richest source of omega-3 fats.
- Canned salmon, sardines, mackerel and, to a lesser extent, tuna are all rich sources of omega-3s; look for canned fish packed in water, sauce or brine, and drain well.
- Fresh fish with higher levels of omega-3s are: Atlantic salmon and smoked salmon; Atlantic, Pacific and Spanish mackerel; sea mullet; southern bluefin tuna; and swordfish. Eastern and Pacific oysters and squid (calamari) are also rich sources.

Mercury in fish

Due to the risk of high levels of mercury in certain species of fish, FSANZ advises limiting them in your diet to one serve per week, eating no other fish in that week. They are billfish (swordfish, broadbill and marlin), shark (flake), orange roughy (also sold as sea perch) and catfish.

Pregnant women, women planning pregnancy and young children should limit their intake of shark (flake), broadbill, marlin and swordfish to no more than one serve per fortnight with no other fish to be consumed during that fortnight. For orange roughy and catfish, the advice is as for the general population—one serve per week, with no other fish being consumed that week.

6 Eat lean red meats, poultry and eggs

Why?

Again, these foods do not have a GI because they are protein food, not a carbohydrate. Red meat is the best source of iron (the nutrient used for carrying oxygen in our blood) you can get.

Good iron status can increase energy levels and improve our exercise tolerance. While adequate iron can be obtained from a vegetarian diet, women particularly must select foods carefully to prevent iron deficiency. A chronic shortage of iron leads to anaemia with symptoms including pale skin, excessive tiredness, breathlessness, irritability and decreased attention span.

How much?

We suggest eating lean meat two or three times a week, and accompanying it with a salad or vegetables. One hundred grams of lean edible meat as part of a balanced diet will meet the daily nutrient needs of an adult, but larger amounts can also be part of a healthy diet. A couple of eggs or 120 grams of skinless chicken provide options for variety once or twice a week.

7 Eat low-fat dairy products

Why?

Milk, cheese, ice-cream, yoghurt, buttermilk and custard are the richest sources of calcium in our diet. Calcium is vital in many body functions so if we don't get enough in our diet, the body will draw it out of our bones. This bone loss over a number of years may lead to osteoporosis and loss of height, curvature of the spine and periodontal disease (deterioration of bones supporting the teeth). By replacing full-fat dairy foods with reduced fat, low-fat or fat-free versions you will reduce your saturated fat intake and actually boost your calcium intake. Plus, new research shows that calcium and other components in dairy play a vital role in fat burning.

How much?

To meet calcium requirements, experts recommend that adults eat two to three servings of dairy products every day. Good low-fat dairy choices include skim, no fat or low-fat milk and no fat or low-fat yoghurts. A serve is a cup of milk (250 ml), 40 grams of cheese or 200 grams of yoghurt.

If you're lactose intolerant, you can still eat yoghurt and cheese. You can also try lactose-reduced milk, high-calcium soy milk, salmon (canned, with bones), high-calcium tofu, calcium-fortified breakfast cereal and dried figs—all great tasting non-dairy sources of calcium.

Milk (GI 27)

Milk is a rich source of protein and vitamin B2 (riboflavin). As whole milk is also a rich source of saturated fat, choose low fat and no-fat milk and milk products. The surprisingly low GI of milk is a combination of the moderate GI of the lactose (milk sugar) plus the effect of the milk protein, which forms a soft curd in the stomach and slows down the rate of stomach emptying.

Yoghurt (GI 19–50)

Yoghurt is rich in calcium, riboflavin and protein. Low-fat natural yoghurt provides the most calcium for the fewest kilojoules. The combination of yoghurt's acidity and high protein contributes to its low GI. Fruit yoghurts made with a sugar-sweetened fruit syrup have a GI of around 33, whereas artificially sweetened yoghurts have a GI of around 14.

Low fat ice-cream (GI 37–49)

Low-fat ice-cream is a delicious source of all the goodies found in milk. It is important that you choose a low-fat (less than 3 grams of fat per 100 grams) variety for regular consumption so that you don't overdo your saturated fat intake. Save the gourmet varieties for an occasional indulgence. Ice-cream has a slightly higher GI than milk because of the presence of sucrose and glucose in addition to lactose.

Chapter 3

The Low GI Diet 12-week Weight-loss Plan

DURING THE '12-WEEK WEIGHT-LOSS PLAN', WE TAKE YOU BY THE hand advising you what to eat and do to get those kilos moving and help you make good eating habits and physical activity a natural part of your life. To help you achieve this, we ask you to focus on three goals each week:

- *The food goal* is designed to make you aware of your current eating patterns and behaviour. It will help you identify areas where you can make changes for the better and includes practical tips for putting the seven dietary guidelines of a low-GI diet into practice so that healthy eating simply becomes a way of life.

- *The exercise goal* includes a combination of aerobic and resistance exercises to increase your fat-burning muscle and tone your body.

- *The activity goal* will show you ways to build more physical activity into your daily life. The single most important difference between long-term weight losers and weight gainers is the amount of activity that they build into their day.

About the menu plans

Each week's sample menu is designed to illustrate appropriate food and meal choices to help you achieve a balanced low-GI diet. You may like to use them simply for ideas, varying them according to your tastes using the simple guidelines for creating balanced low-GI meals on pages 188–91. Don't expect to follow them exactly, particularly in the early weeks. As your habits change, your diet may more closely reflect the menus.

How much food is right for you?

We don't give you specific quantities of food in the menus. One restricted energy diet can't fit all because each one of us has different energy requirements that are affected by things such as how active we are, our size, how much muscle we have, whether we have a sedentary job or a physically demanding one etc. Your aim is to eat just a little less than your body needs so your body has to dig into those fat stores to make up the deficit.

In this chapter we provide you with the choice of 10 different weight-based energy levels (5 for men and 5 for women). See page 45.

All you do is select the right energy level for you based on your current weight (Step 1). This will give you the number of daily serves you need of carb-rich foods, protein-rich foods and the good fats to make sure that you lose weight at a rate that's appropriate for you and maximises your engine revs during weight loss (Step 2).

Whatever your energy level, everyone needs to eat at least five serves of vegetables and two serves of fruit every day. Higher energy levels could have more. Here's how you do it:

Step 1: Identify the energy level that corresponds to your current weight.

Women		Men	
Weight (kg)	**Energy level**	**Weight (kg)**	**Energy level**
less than 70	1	less than 90	6
71–80	2	91–100	7
81–90	3	101–110	8
91–100	4	111–120	9
greater than 100	5	greater than 120	10

Step 2: Highlight the row that corresponds to your energy level—this gives you the recommended number of daily serves of each food type.

	Recommended number of daily serves		
Energy level	**Carb-rich foods**	**Protein-rich foods**	**Fat-rich foods**
1	6	4	2
2	8	5	2
3	10	5	3
4	12	6	3
5	14	7	3
6	16	8	4
7	18	9	4
8	20	10	4
9	22	11	5
10	24	12	6

Step 3: Plus five serves of vegetables and two serves of fruit every day.

Serving sizes

1 serve of vegetables   ×5

½ cup (75 g) cooked vegetables (other than potato, sweet
   potato and corn)

1 cup raw/salad vegetables

1 cup vegetable soup or juice

---

1 serve of fruit   ×2

1 medium piece or 2 small pieces (150 g) fresh fruit

1½ tablespoons sultanas, 4–5 dried apricots/figs/prunes (30
   g dried fruit)

½ cup (125 ml) fruit juice

1 cup diced or canned fruit

×6 #### Carb-rich foods: 1 serve provides 15–20 g
carbohydrate

1 slice bread

½ cup (30 g) processed breakfast cereal

¼ cup raw oats or muesli

⅓ cup cooked rice or other small grains such as cracked
   wheat (bulgur), couscous, barley

½ cup cooked pasta or noodles

2 small potatoes or half a medium sweet potato (100 g)

½ cup corn or ½ large ear of corn

½ cup cooked legumes (dried beans, chickpeas) (can also
   count as ½ protein serve)

x4 **Protein-rich foods: 1 serve provides 10–15 g protein**

50 g raw lean meat, poultry, fish or seafood

3 slices (60 g) ham/pastrami/deli-sliced meat

50 g canned fish, drained

1 cup skim milk

200 g carton low-fat yoghurt

1 cup beans or chickpeas (can also count as 2 carb-rich serves)

100 g tofu

2 eggs

---

x2 **Fat-rich foods: 1 serve provides 10 g fat**

2 teaspoons (10 ml) oils

1–2 tablespoons oil and vinegar dressing

2 teaspoons (10 g) margarine/butter

3 teaspoons (15 g) reduced-fat spread

3 teaspoons peanut butter*

30 g raw nuts or seeds*

¼ (50 g) avocado

2 tablespoons (40 g) reduced-fat cream cheese*

40 g (2 pre-packed slices) reduced-fat hard cheese*

30 g regular cheese*

---

*These foods are also good sources of protein, but have a particularly high fat content.

How to apply your energy level to a daily menu

Fiona and Dave both need to lose some weight. Fiona currently weighs 76 kilograms and is aiming to lose 6 kilograms over the 12-week Weight-loss Plan. Dave weighs in at 115 kilograms and is looking to lose about the same amount for starters—and keep it off. They want to be able to enjoy their meals together and on the Weight-loss Plan they can. Here's how.

According to the tables on page 45, Fiona is on level 2 and should be aiming to include eight serves of carb-rich foods, four serves of protein-rich foods and two serves of fat-rich foods in addition to her five servings of vegetables and two of fruit each day.

If Dave ate the same amount as Fiona, he would be ravenously hungry and unlikely to stick with the Weight-loss Plan for long. All he needs to do is change the quantities of foods, sometimes adding extra foods for his size and energy requirements. Using the tables Dave sees that he is on energy level 9 and should be aiming to include 22 serves of carb-rich foods, 11 serves of protein-rich foods and five serves of fat-rich foods a day plus at least five servings of vegetables and two of fruit.

Fiona's day at a glance

	Vegetables	Fruit	Carb-rich foods	Protein-rich foods	Fat-rich foods
Breakfast: ½ cup muesli with ½ cup skim milk and a handful of sliced strawberries		1	2	½	
Lunch: 1 cup of tomato soup with a sandwich of 2 slices grainy bread with 3 slices ham, 1 cup salad vegies, flavoured with mustard	2		2	1	
Dinner: 100 g grilled salmon served with a cob of corn, ½ cup mixed bean salsa, 2 cups green salad and 1 tablespoon olive oil and vinegar dressing	2		3	2	1
Snacks: 1 cup fruit salad topped with ½ carton low-fat yoghurt and ¼ cup crunchy muesli		1	1	½	
30 g almonds and 1 cup of vegetable juice	1				1
TOTALS	**5**	**2**	**8**	**4**	**2**

Fiona's eight serves of carbohydrate come from:

- ½ cup muesli (2 serves) at breakfast
- 2 slices bread (2) at lunchtime
- 1 corn cob (2) and ½ cup bean salsa (1) at dinner
- ¼ cup crunchy muesli (1) for snacks

Her four serves of protein come from:

- ½ cup skim milk (½) at breakfast
- 3 slices ham (1) at lunchtime
- 100 grams salmon (2) at dinner
- Half a carton yoghurt (½) as a snack

Her two serves of fat come from:

- 1 tablespoon oil and vinegar dressing (1) at dinner (mix equal portions of oil and vinegar)
- 30 grams almonds (1) as a snack

This day provides 5800 kilojoules, 85 grams of protein, 166 grams of carbohydrate, 40 grams of fat and 35 grams of fibre.

Dave's day at a glance

	Vegetables	Fruit	Carb-rich foods	Protein-rich foods	Fat-rich foods
Breakfast: 1 cup muesli with 1 cup skim milk and a handful of sliced strawberries		1	4	1	

	Vegetables	Fruit	Carb-rich foods	Protein-rich foods	Fat-rich foods
2 boiled eggs with 2 slices grainy toast spread with 2 teaspoons butter/ margarine			2	1	1
Lunch: 1 cup tomato soup with 2 sandwiches of 4 slices grainy bread with 6 slices of ham, 2 cups salad vegies, flavoured with mustard	3		4	2	
Dinner: 200 g salmon grilled served with 2 cobs of corn, 1 cup mixed bean salsa, 3 cups green salad and 2 tablespoons dressing	3		6	4	2
Snacks: 1 cup fruit salad topped with 1 carton low-fat yoghurt and ½ cup crunchy muesli		1	2	1	
2 grainy muffins topped with baked beans			4	1	
60 g almonds and a fruit smoothie made with 1 cup skim milk		1		1	2
TOTALS	**6**	**3**	**22**	**11**	**5**

Dave's 22 serves of carbohydrate come from:
- 1 cup muesli (4) and 2 slices toast (2) at breakfast
- 4 slices of bread (4) at lunchtime
- 2 corn cobs (4), 1 cup bean salsa (2) at dinner
- 2 grainy muffins (4) as a snack
- ½ cup crunchy muesli (2) as a snack

His 11 serves of protein come from:
- 1 cup skim milk (1) and 2 boiled eggs (1) for breakfast
- 6 slices lean ham (2) for lunch
- 200 grams grilled salmon (4) for dinner
- 1 carton low-fat yoghurt (1), 1 cup baked beans (1) and a smoothie made with 1 cup skim milk (1) as snacks

His five serves of fat come from:
- 2 teaspoons of margarine on his toast for breakfast (1)
- 2 tablespoons of olive oil and vinegar dressing on his salad at dinner (2) (mix equal portions of oil and vinegar)
- 60 grams almonds as a snack (2)

Dave's typical day has similar proportions of energy from protein, fat and carbohydrate, but larger quantities of each, providing 12 800 kilojoules, 190 grams of protein, 100 grams of fat, 348 grams of carbohydrate and 69 grams of fibre.

Of course, as you lose weight you may find that you move down an energy level—this is because with less weight to move around, your energy requirements also fall. Re-evaluate how much you should be eating every month to ensure the best success in reaching your goals.

Do you prefer to let appetite be your guide?

While we suggest that most people start off by measuring their serving sizes according to the previous tables, some prefer a less structured approach. If this sounds like you, you may be able to use your appetite as the best indicator of how much food you need. To ensure your meals are correctly balanced, follow these three simple steps when planning meals:

1   *Start* with your low-GI carbohydrate.
2   *Add* a generous serve of vegetables and/or fruit.
3   *Plus* some protein for good measure with a little healthy fat if you wish.

About the exercise plans

To gain the most benefit from the exercises outlined in the plan you need to work at an appropriate intensity—if the exercise feels too easy, you are not maximising your energy expenditure or the amount of fat burnt to fuel the exercise; if you try too hard you will struggle to keep going for the allocated time, you will find it uncomfortable and unenjoyable, and you are unlikely to keep it up on a regular basis.

You don't need fancy equipment such as heart rate monitors to measure your exercise intensity—all you need is a simple scale of how you feel. The Perceived Rate of Exertion (PRE) scale has been used for years by fitness instructors to guide their clients in their workouts. We will use a modified version of this scale to help you to maximise your fat loss and energy expenditure at each workout session. As you are exercising, ask yourself, on a scale of 1 to 10, how you are feeling, using the following table as a guide.

The PRE Scale

FOR HEALTH	**1**	At rest
	2	Minimal exertion
	3	Comfortable and could easily continue for some time
	4	Starting to get a little breathless but relatively comfortable
FOR FITNESS	**5**	A little breathless and can feel heart rate elevated
	6	Breathing harder, heart rate elevated but can still talk comfortably
	7	Breathing hard, exercise much more difficult and cannot maintain for more than a few minutes
FOR PERFORMANCE	**8**	Much more intense and difficult to maintain, can only keep going at this intensity for a short time
	9	Extremely intense exercise, cannot talk comfortably and breathing hard
	10	Maximum intensity which can only be maintained for a few seconds

The good news is that during the 12-week plan you will never be working above level 5. This means you will never need to experience intense or uncomfortable exercise. Levels of intensity above 5 are useful for people such as athletes who need to stretch their fitness levels to the extreme in order to improve their performance in their sport. Thankfully, if you are seeking the health benefits of exercise and aiming to lose body fat, working at the lower, more comfortable levels will better help you to reach your goals. In fact, in the early days of the program, you are going to be sticking to a PRE level of 3–4, the perfect level to improve your health and get you burning fat. As you progress and become fitter, we incorporate short sessions at level 5. This will help you to keep your weight under control for a lifetime as your body becomes a far more efficient fat-burning machine.

The exercise involved in the Weight-loss Plan incorporates both aerobic and resistance training:

- **Aerobic training** is any movement that gets you breathing a little harder—by definition, aerobic means 'using oxygen'. This sort of exercise works your heart and lungs and burns energy, helping you to increase your daily energy expenditure and burn body fat. We have opted to use walking as our aerobic exercise but cycling, running, swimming, aerobics, rowing and stepping are all good forms of aerobic exercise.

- **Resistance training** is any exercise that makes your muscles work against a resistance. This includes lifting weights, using resistance bands or simply using your own body weight as resistance. This sort of exercise is crucial to strengthen muscles, achieve and maintain good posture and tone your body. In addition, by building a little more lean muscle mass you increase your metabolic rate. As muscle is far more metabolically active than fat, the more muscle mass you have, the more energy you burn all of the time. To achieve fat loss and maintain that fat loss, resistance training offers great advantages and is an invaluable part of the Weight-loss Plan.

At the start of each week, get out your diary and schedule in an exact time for all your walks and workouts. If you leave it to happen spontaneously, the week will be over before you know it and you won't have started. Treat each exercise session as any other appointment and stick to it—if you have to postpone a session, make sure you reschedule it for another time. With the walking sessions, you have the option of breaking the walk into two shorter walks if you don't have enough time all at once. You could try doing ten minutes of walking first thing in the morning and the rest in the evening.

You won't need any specialist equipment. Simply wear comfortable, loose clothing and supportive walking shoes— trainers are perfect, or use any comfortable, supportive shoe you have.

While it is commonly thought that moving more quickly makes exercise harder, the opposite is in fact true for resistance exercise. To gain the best results from the resistance exercises, move slowly and focus on getting your technique spot-on. Try counting in seconds, taking two seconds to get to the end position and two seconds to get back to the start.

Remember that *anything* you do more than you are currently doing is a step in the right direction. Use the exercise plan as a guide and do as much as you can. If the weeks are progressing too quickly for you, simply stick with the same plan for a few more weeks, moving on to the next week's plan once you feel ready.

The resistance exercises may not be suitable for those with limiting injuries or conditions such as arthritis. If you feel pain at any time, you should stop the exercise. Consult a qualified personal trainer for an individualised program—see page 212.

Week 1

Are you ready to begin? For this first week, focus on the following goals:

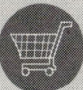

FOOD GOAL

Increase your awareness of what you eat and why.

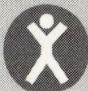

EXERCISE GOAL

Aim to walk at a steady, comfortable pace for a total of 20 minutes on four days. *Plus* complete the two resistance exercises outlined on three days.

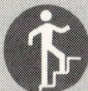

ACTIVITY GOAL

Rather than standing still on escalators and moving walkways, keep moving and walk to the end.

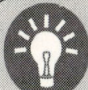

FOOD FOR THOUGHT

What is the GI of your diet?

> **FOOD GOAL**
>
> Increase your awareness of what you eat and why.

Your first dietary goal with the Weight-loss Plan is to keep a food diary to identify exactly what you usually eat and why you make the choices you do. You may think you already know what you eat, but there is nothing like writing it down to increase your awareness of all that you eat and drink.

Looking back over the record at the end of the week will enable you to compare your eating habits with the low-GI diet food choices (see Chapter 2) and serving sizes (see pages 44–47), and help you identify foods that you could substitute or minimise. A food diary can also reveal links between what you eat and the mood, environment or situations you find yourself in—we look at alleviating problem areas next week.

- Try to keep a diary, just for one week. You can keep it for longer if you wish, but it can become tedious and ends up being incomplete. One complete week is better than three sketchy weeks.
- Choose a normal week in your life—one that is representative of most weeks (not one where you are away on holidays, for example).
- Use a small notebook that you can take everywhere and write down everything you eat and drink as soon as possible after you have eaten it (or while you are eating it). Note where you are, what you are doing and how you feel.

You can also use the diary to write down your physical activity. We have included a template for your diary on page 184.

EXERCISE GOAL

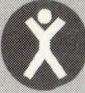

Aim to walk at a steady, comfortable pace for a total of 20 minutes on four days. *Plus* complete the two resistance exercises outlined on three days.

Walking

Using the PRE scale on page 54, aim to walk at about level 3—this means you should feel comfortable at all times and be able to carry out a conversation while walking. You should feel warmer as the blood flow around the body increases, taking fuel to your working muscles—this means you are burning more fat and increasing your daily energy expenditure.

Resistance exercises

Lower body exercises	Upper body exercises	'Core' strength abdominals and back
Squats 2 sets of 10		Leg extensions 10 each leg

NEW EXERCISES

Squats

The squat is arguably the best lower body exercise you can do. The muscles of your thighs and bottom are the biggest muscle group in the body and this means exercises involving these muscles use the most energy—exactly what you want to help you lose body fat.

Strengthens and tones: thighs and bottom

How to do it:

1 Stand with your feet parallel and just wider than hip-distance apart. Extend your arms directly in front of you at chest height, with hands clasped.

2 Lengthen your spine by standing tall and pulling in your belly below the navel to support the lower back.

3 Imagine you have a chair behind you and sit back until you 'touch' the imaginary chair. As you sit back, make sure you keep your arms parallel to the floor and your chest 'proud'.

4 Squeeze your bottom muscles and push your heels into the floor to get back to the standing position.

Remember: Throughout the exercise, keep your weight on the back two-thirds of your feet: you should be able to wiggle your toes. One last thing—don't forget to breathe normally.

How many: 2 sets of 10 with a short rest in between

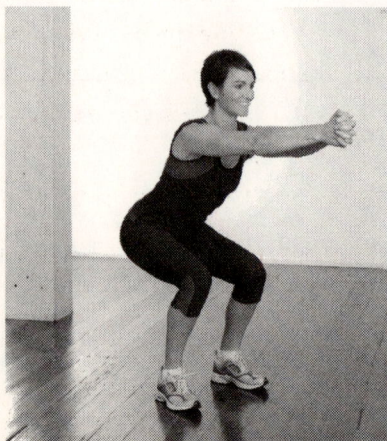

Single leg extensions

One of the most important groups of muscles for you to exercise are those involved in posture and back support. (These are the deep abdominal muscles that lie below the sixpack of stomach muscles you can see on the very lean men seen advertising unnecessary abdominal trainer machines.) They lie across your body and act like a belt, holding in your waist to provide support, particularly for the lower back. By working this group of muscles you develop core strength that will immediately improve your posture (making you look slimmer), reduce the risk of back pain and strengthen you from the inside out.

Strengthens and tones: the 'core' (deep abdominals)

How to do it:
1 Lie flat on your back on the floor with your knees bent in towards your chest, and arms by your sides with hands flat to the floor.
2 Pull in your belly as if trying to shorten the distance between your navel and spine—it should feel as if you are bracing the abdominal wall. Extend one leg out parallel to the floor while keeping the abdominals braced.
3 Bring the leg back in and repeat on the other side.

Remember: Breathe normally (it's easy to hold your breath subconsciously during this exercise).

How many: 20 (10 on each leg)

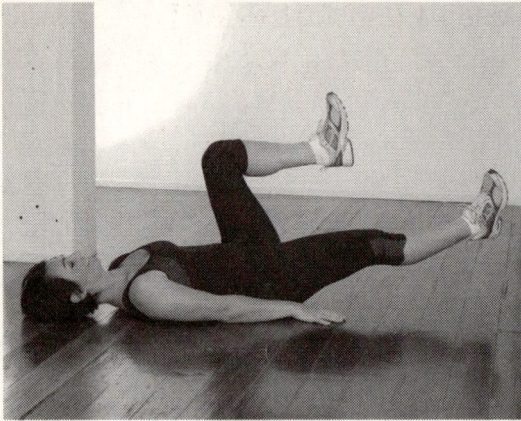

Sample diary

Monday	Tuesday	Wednesday	Thursday	Friday	Saturday	Sunday
	20 min walk		20 min walk		20 min walk	20 min walk
	+ resistance exercises		+ resistance exercises		+ resistance exercises	
	25 mins		25 mins		25 mins	20 mins

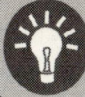

FOOD FOR THOUGHT

What is the GI of your diet?

Using the information from your food diary, answer the quiz below to gain a clearer idea of where you need to make changes to lower the GI of your diet.

QUIZ: What is the GI of your diet?

Simply circle the option that most closely matches your usual diet.

1 The type of bread I most often eat is

a a grainy low-GI variety

b sourdough or 'health' loaf

c regular white or wholemeal sandwich bread

3 I eat 2 or more different pieces of fruit

a most days

b 3–4 days a week

c 1–2 days a week

5 I eat pasta or noodles

a 2 or more times a week

b once a week

c rarely or never

2 The type of breakfast cereal I usually eat is

a traditional rolled oats, muesli, or a commercial low-GI type

b a higher fibre commercial cereal such as wheat biscuits or flakes

c A low-fibre puffed or flaked cereal

4 I eat legumes (including baked beans, lentils, chickpeas, kidney beans, salad beans, etc.) or barley

a 2 or more times a week

b once a week

c rarely or never

6 I eat lower GI forms of potato and/ or sweetcorn instead of regular potato

a 2 or more times a week

b once a week

c rarely or never

7 Of the following serves of food: I would eat at least 2 serves
- 1 cup milk (any type)
- 1 cup yoghurt (any type)
- ½ cup custard
- 2 scoops low-fat ice-cream

a   most days

b   3–4 days a week

c   1–2 days a week or less

Your score card:

Score 1 point for each time you answered (**a**)

Score 2 points for each time you answered (**b**)

Score 3 points for each time you answered (**c**)

If your total was:

7–10   Well done—your diet is likely to have a low GI. The carbohydrate foods you have indicated you eat most frequently are low-GI choices. You may still need to consider serving sizes to facilitate weight loss. Keep reading because there is lots more to a healthy low-GI diet than low-GI foods alone.

11–17   Your diet is likely to have an intermediate GI. This is the same as the average diet of most people in Western countries. You have indicated that you eat a mixture of low, medium and possibly high-GI carbohydrate choices, and, while variety is good, high-GI foods may be hindering your efforts at weight loss. Choosing more foods that fit option (a) will reduce the GI of your diet.

18–21 Your diet is likely to have a high GI. Many of your carbohydrate choices have high GI values, increasing your insulin demand and keeping your body in a state that favours fat storage. In order to lose weight it will be beneficial to swap at least half of your high-GI carb foods for those with a low GI. Choosing more foods that fit option (a) will reduce the GI of your diet.

Week 1 Menu Plan

	BREAKFAST	SNACK	
MONDAY	Grainy toast with peanut butter (no butter) and a glass of fruit or vegetable juice	Canned fruit snack pack	
TUESDAY	Grainy toast with low-fat cheese	A banana	
WEDNESDAY	Low-fat milk coffee or hot chocolate with raisin toast	Dried fruit and nut mix	
THURSDAY	Natural muesli with low-fat milk, topped with fruit and no fat yoghurt	A banana	
FRIDAY	High-fibre cereal with low-fat milk and fruit	An apple	
SATURDAY	Sautéed mushrooms with parsley and shallots, low-GI toast and a poached egg	A mandarin	
SUNDAY	A boiled egg, lean bacon, tomato, mushrooms and baked beans, and a glass of vegetable juice	Small fruit smoothie	

LUNCH	SNACK	DINNER
Sourdough rye with roast beef, horseradish, sliced tomato and snowpea sprouts	Reduced-fat cheddar cheese with an apple and grainy crackers	Baked white fish fillets with chopped parsley. Serve with chopped spinach and lemon, yellow squash, carrots and a couple of baby new potatoes. Low-fat yoghurt
Tuna, celery, onion, tomato and olives tossed in balsamic vinaigrette with lettuce and grainy crackers	Low-fat yoghurt	Vegetable Frittata (see page 225) and tossed salad. Baked apple and low-fat custard
Avocado, chicken and lettuce wrap	Fresh fruit	Lean steak with mushrooms, sweet potato mash, green beans and zucchini
Salad with lettuce, celery, apple, walnuts, mayonnaise and tuna	Low-fat ice-cream in a cone	Tuna with canned tomatoes, artichoke quarters, kalamata olives, garlic, sliced zucchini and tomato paste tossed through spiral pasta
Chinese combination long soup	Low-fat yoghurt	Pork and vegetable (broccoli, carrot, capsicum and onion) stir-fry with cashew nuts and Doongara CleverRice
Toasted soy and linseed English muffins spread with creamed corn, sliced fresh mushrooms and a sprinkle of grated cheese, heated under the grill	Oatmeal biscuits	Lamb roast with mint sauce, baked sweet potato, pumpkin, onion and steamed peas, beans and cauliflower. Fresh fruit salad
Thai beef salad made with lean beef strips, mixed salad greens and a dressing of chilli, garlic, lime juice, brown sugar and Thai fish sauce, sprinkled with cellophane noodles	A small handful of almonds	Minestrone soup. A low-fat yoghurt and fruit

Week 2

Being overweight is *not* about lacking willpower, and if you have ever been on a diet you will know that to be the case. Changing habits that are ingrained in our daily lives is extremely difficult and takes time (about a year to be exact!). Through Week 1 the focus was on becoming more aware of what you eat and starting to incorporate more low-GI foods in your diet. This week we help you pinpoint your bad habits and set goals that will lead you towards healthier habits. Your goals to work on this week are:

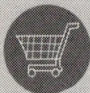

FOOD GOAL

Pinpoint your bad habits and set three SMART food goals.

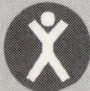

EXERCISE GOAL

Aim to walk at a steady, comfortable pace for 20 minutes on four days. *Plus* complete the three resistance exercises outlined on three days.

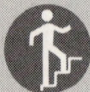

ACTIVITY GOAL

For all short journeys that would take less than five minutes in the car, walk instead.

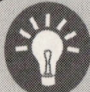

FOOD FOR THOUGHT

Time for a change.

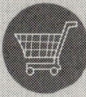

FOOD GOAL

Pinpoint your bad habits and set three SMART food goals.

Having put in the effort and recorded your eating patterns last week, you now have the opportunity to identify the eating habits that you're going to change. Making changes begins with setting goals. Ideally your goals should be **S**pecific, **M**easurable, **A**chievable, **R**ealistic and **T**ime-specific.

For example, it is unrealistic to set the goal 'I'll stop eating chocolate' and may be unachievable to say 'I will take my lunch from home every day'. These all-or-nothing goals tend to set us up for failure and are not helpful in achieving long-term changes.

Examples of SMART goals in these instances:
- I will allow myself a 75 g chocolate bar once a week.
- I will start preparing my own lunch to take to work on Mondays and Tuesdays.

Habits that you want to change may also relate to your eating behaviour. The following checklist is to help you identify problem eating behaviours. Referring back to your food diary if you need to, tick off any of the following that are regular events for you.

❐ Too many snacks
❐ Irregular meals
❐ Nibbling all day
❐ Eat while watching television
❐ Eat when preparing food

☐   Serve or am served more than I need, but eat it anyway

☐   Impulse-buy unplanned foods

☐   Eat when not hungry, but because I'm either bored, tired, depressed or angry

☐   Eat out too often

☐   Eat when driving or travelling

☐   Eat too fast

☐   Linger at the table, eating more even though I'm satisfied

☐   Go back for seconds

☐   Overeat night snacks

☐   Always finish plate even if I feel full

☐   Drink too much alcohol

☐   Buy foods for the family that I don't intend eating, but can't resist

Now, given your checklist of problem eating behaviours and your food diary, select two or three of your eating habits or food choices that you would like to change and brainstorm possible solutions.

Set yourself three goals relating to what or how you eat. Remember, your goals must be relevant to you and your situation, and should be specific, measurable, achievable, realistic and time-specific. Commit to these goals, trying to adhere to them as much as you can. At the end of the week, think about how successful you were in sticking to your goal. Did it work for you? Are you willing to keep it going? If the answer is no, then try setting another goal, based on a different solution to your habits and keep experimenting until you find the change that works for you.

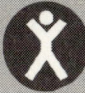

EXERCISE GOAL

Aim to walk at a steady, comfortable pace for 20 minutes on four days. *Plus* complete the three resistance exercises outlined on three days.

Resistance exercises

Lower body exercises	Upper body exercises	'Core' strength abdominals and back
Squats 2 sets of 10	Assisted push-ups 2 sets of 10	Leg extensions 10 each leg

NEW EXERCISE

Assisted push-ups

The push-up is undeniably one of the best upper body exercises you can do. The push-up involves the muscles of the chest, shoulders and arms and is therefore an efficient means of toning the upper body all at once.

Why do most people hate push-ups? The answer is easy—because they are hard! In fact, they are even harder if you are carrying too much body weight since you are effectively lifting your own body weight against gravity. Here is a modified version of the traditional push-up, which enables you to gain the benefits of the exercise but makes it easier for you to perform it correctly. You will need a low coffee table—alternatively, use the second or third bottom step of a set of stairs.

Strengthens and tones: chest, shoulders and arms

How to do it:

1 Start in a kneeling position with your hands wider than your shoulders on the edge of the table/stair. Move your knees back until your body is a straight diagonal line from head to knee.

2 Slowly lower your chest towards the edge of the table/stair while keeping your back flat and without letting your bottom stick up.

3 At the bottom of the move, your elbows should be directly above your hands—adjust your hand position as appropriate before returning slowly to the starting position.

How many: 2 sets of 10 repetitions with a short rest in between

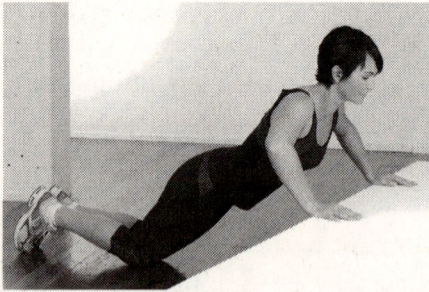

Sample diary

Monday	Tuesday	Wednesday	Thursday	Friday	Saturday	Sunday
	20 min walk		20 min walk		20 min walk	20 min walk
	+ resistance exercises		+ resistance exercises		+ resistance exercises	
	25 mins		25 mins		25 mins	20 mins

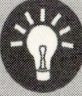

FOOD FOR THOUGHT
Time for a change.

The fact that you are reading this very page suggests that you are at least *contemplating* making some changes to the way you eat. People don't make changes instantaneously; they work their way up to it gradually, often going through definable stages. A description of the stages of change in relation to our eating habits looks like this:

Pre-contemplation

At this stage you're not thinking about changing your eating habits; what you're doing is appropriate for *you* at this time in your life. You could read this book and then put it away for later reference.

↓

Contemplation

Now you're beginning to think about change but just haven't got around to it. Weigh up the benefits and costs of making a change. If the benefits outweigh the costs, then you're ready to move on to preparation.

↓

Preparation

Now you have decided to change and are preparing to do so. Attempting change without prior planning makes relapse more likely. So, ask yourself, what do you think you can change?

↓

Action

You are now actually in the throes of making changes to the way you eat. Your goals ought to be **SMART—Specific, Measurable, Achievable, Realistic** and **Time-specific,** for example:

- Every two days buy four nice pieces of fresh fruit to eat.
- Buy and use only fat-reduced milk for the next month as a trial.

Your goals must be relevant to you and your situation, so checking back through your food diary could be a good place from which to plan your behaviour changes.

↓

Maintenance

At this point you're committed to maintaining your changes and have no desire to return to your old ways. You face relapses every so often but getting through them will lead to your changes becoming your new healthy habits.

Identifying at which stage you are currently should help you move forward to the next stage.

At what stage of change are you?
Circle the answer that best fits you and identify the stage you are at using the key opposite.

Have you been trying to lose weight?

a Yes, I have been making changes to my diet and exercise for at least 3 months.

b Yes, I have been trying to lose weight within the last 3 months.

c No, but I intend to make a start.

d No, and I do not intend to at the moment.

Key: Answer (**a**) = maintenance stage

Answer (**b**) = action stage

Answer (**c**) = contemplation/preparation stage

Answer (**d**) = pre-contemplation stage

A word of warning: change can be difficult and changing the way you eat is no exception. Even with all the good will in the world, celebrations, cheesecakes, cravings, nights out or chocolate will always be lurking around the corner just waiting to test your resolve. It might help to bear in mind that normal, healthy eating includes all foods, and 'lapses' are just a normal part of change.

Our tips for approaching dietary change

1 Aim to make changes gradually. Acknowledge your stage of change.

2 Attempt the easiest changes first. Nothing inspires like success!

3 Break big changes into a number of smaller changes.

4 Accept lapses in your habits as a characteristic of being human.

If you feel like you need some extra help in changing the way you eat, seek out professional assistance from an accredited practising dietitian (APD). (Visit www.daa.asn.au or call 1800 812 942 in Australia or www.dietitians.org.nz in New Zealand to find a dietitian.)

Week 2 Menu Plan

	BREAKFAST	SNACK
MONDAY	Fruit loaf lightly spread with ricotta cheese and jam	An apple and a few almonds
TUESDAY	Multigrain English muffin with scrambled egg and a tomato juice	2 kiwi fruit
WEDNESDAY	Grainy toast with hazelnut spread and an apple	Small handful of unsalted nuts
THURSDAY	Low-fat vanilla yoghurt with sliced fresh nectarine and strawberries, topped with muesli	An Apricot and Almond Cookie (see page 263)
FRIDAY	Low-GI cereal topped with sliced pears, low-fat milk and a freshly squeezed orange juice	2 ginger nut biscuits
SATURDAY	Lean grilled bacon with sliced tomato on grainy toast	A low-fat fruit yoghurt
SUNDAY	Porridge with a garnish of frozen or fresh berries, low-fat natural yoghurt and a sprinkle of brown sugar	A slice of raisin toast

LUNCH	SNACK	DINNER
Ham and salad grainy roll, skim milk latte	Wedge of melon	Moroccan-style Lentil and Vegetable Stew with Couscous (see page 255)
Greek salad with low-fat feta and olives and a small grainy roll	Some low-fat ice-cream	Tandoori chicken with Basmati rice, lentil dhal and cucumber raita plus a mango lassi
Toasted sourdough with avocado, sliced tomato and grilled lean bacon or double smoked ham	Fresh orange quarters	Lamb shish kebabs with garlic and tahini sauce served with tabbouli and pieces of flatbread
Garden salad with sliced chicken breast	Fresh pear	Spinach and ricotta cannelloni with pine nuts and tomato sauce. Serve with a mixed green salad with vinaigrette
Wholemeal Lebanese bread with shaved ham, grated carrot, shredded lettuce, sliced tomato, low-fat grated cheese and mayonnaise	Fruit salad	Cook a whole fish, such as snapper, by wrapping in two layers of foil and cook on the barbecue for 25–30 minutes. Serve with roasted sweet potato wedges
Tuna, onion, lettuce and cheese on a grainy roll	Fruit and nut mix	Prawn and Mango Salad with Chilli Lime Dressing (see page 253). A wedge of melon with a scoop of low-fat ice-cream
Tacos topped with Mexican beans, diced tomato, shredded lettuce, avocado and grated reduced-fat cheese	An apple	Barbecued steak with roast vegetable salad and green salad

Week 3

Unless you have diabetes and are diligent about testing your blood glucose levels, you are probably completely unaware of your own fluctuations over the course of a day. Yet this can have a major effect on what, how much and when you eat, as well as whether you store or burn body fat. This week, focus on these goals:

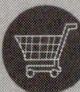

FOOD GOAL

Minimise your blood glucose fluctuations by getting the smart carbs going.

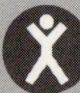

EXERCISE GOAL

Aim to walk at a steady, comfortable pace (level 3 on the PRE scale) for a total of 20 minutes on five days. *Plus* complete the four resistance exercises on three days.

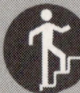

ACTIVITY GOAL

Arrange a social activity for the weekend that does not involve food or drink, but something active instead. Why not try going to the golf driving range, cycling in the park or ten-pin bowling with a bunch of friends.

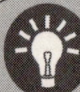

FOOD FOR THOUGHT

Why your blood glucose level is so important.

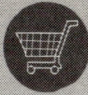

> **FOOD GOAL**
>
> Minimise your blood glucose fluctuations by getting the smart carbs going.

Want to keep your engine running smoothly all day? Then *slow release* low-GI smart carbs are the ones for you. The slow digestion of low-GI carbs trickles fuel into your system at a steady rate, reducing insulin levels and minimising blood glucose fluctuations. This small change can potentially make a huge difference to your waistline in the long term. It's the starchy carb staples in your diet that have the greatest impact—so check you are eating the right carbs using the following table.

Starchy staples	Minimise these high-GI choices	Use these low-GI varieties instead
The bread you eat	Soft white breads	Sourdough
	Light and airy, smooth-textured white and wholemeal bread	Dense, wholegrain, low-GI breads
	Scones, pikelets, dampers	Low-GI fruit breads
The cereals in your pantry	Refined, commercial processed cereals	Traditional rolled oats, muesli and barley-based cereals
Main meal carbs	Potatoes: mashed, chips and French fries	Almera, Carisma, baby new potatoes, sweet potato, sweetcorn, pasta, noodles, butter beans, lentils, chickpeas
	Jasmine, brown and Arborio rice	Basmati, Doongara CleverRice, Moolgiri rice
The foods you snack on	Light and crispy crackers, doughnuts, pretzels	Fresh or dried fruit, low-fat yoghurt and nuts

BASE YOUR FOOD GOALS THIS WEEK AROUND MAKING YOUR STARCHY STAPLES THE SMART LOW GI TYPES.

> ### EXERCISE GOAL
>
> Aim to walk at a steady, comfortable pace (level 3 on the PRE scale) for a total of 20 minutes on five days. *Plus* complete the four resistance exercises on three days.

Resistance exercises

Lower body exercises	Upper body exercises	'Core' strength abdominals and back
Squats 2 sets of 10	Assisted push-ups 2 sets of 10	Leg extensions 10 each leg
Lunges 10 each leg		

NEW EXERCISE

Lunges

This week we add one more exercise for the lower body. Lunges are a little more difficult than squats because one leg has to work harder. Again, they are very effective at working the thighs and bottom, with the lower leg also doing some work for a complete lower body workout. The most common mistake is to have your feet too close together, which makes it difficult to lunge without bringing your weight forward over the front foot—aim for a long stride and work on keeping the upper body upright with your chest proud. Use a broom handle or the back of a chair to help with balance when you first do this exercise; as you

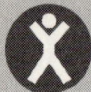

become stronger you will be able to complete the exercise without assistance.

Strengthens: bottom and legs

How to do it:

1 Stand with your feet hip-width apart and then step one foot back in a long stride behind you. Your feet should still be parallel—you should not feel like you are tightrope walking, but in a strong, tall stance.

2 Centre your body weight between your feet and tuck your hips under to maintain a long, strong spine. Slowly drop your body weight down until your front thigh is parallel to the floor and the back knee is under your hip.

3 Push your front heel into the floor to push you back to the top.

Remember: Your back heel should not touch the floor during the exercise—you should be up on the ball of your foot throughout the motion.

How many: 10 lunges on each leg

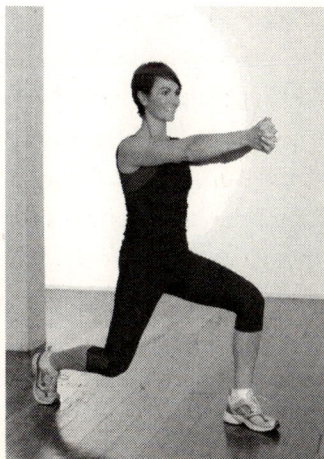

Sample diary

Monday	Tuesday	Wednesday	Thursday	Friday	Saturday	Sunday
20 min walk	20 min walk		20 min walk		20 min walk	20 min walk
	+ resistance exercises		+ resistance exercises		+ resistance exercises	
20 mins	30 mins		30 mins		30 mins	20 mins

'Tomorrow I am running a half marathon and the glycemic index helped get me there!' – Tricia

I am a firm believer in the GI because it has changed my life. I am a runner and I found that as I was training and trying 'fad' diets at the same time, I was getting migraines about once a week. I was really tired all the time and often had a nap in the middle of the day. Then one day I found the GI. I started putting it into practice right away. One of the things I love about the GI is it is so simple. I followed the recommendations for athletes, and ate low glycemic before a workout and higher after. It has not only gotten rid of my headaches, but it has also increased my endurance in running. I feel healthier and I have so much energy. I tell everyone I know about the GI, because it just makes sense to me. It has become a healthy lifestyle for me and my family. Tomorrow I am running a half marathon and the glycemic index helped get me there! Keep up the good work!

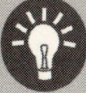

FOOD FOR THOUGHT

Why your blood glucose level is so important.

A normal blood glucose level is the difference between life and death—literally. A low blood glucose level can result in coma and death within minutes. A high blood glucose level will kill you too but the process takes years. If a high blood glucose condition is not treated, it will result in blindness, heart disease and kidney failure. Unless you have diabetes or its predecessor (pre-diabetes), such morbid thoughts won't trouble you. In healthy individuals blood glucose levels are held automatically within a fairly narrow range (between 3 and 10 millimoles per litre). They go up and down when we eat; if we skip a meal (or exclude carbs), the liver draws on its reserves of carbohydrates. When those run out, the liver will make glucose using building blocks from the breakdown of protein and fat stores. The reason for such fine control is that glucose is virtually the sole fuel of our metabolically expensive brain. Without glucose, it shuts down and everything else grinds to a halt, too.

One in four adults (especially those with excess fat around the middle) has undesirably high blood glucose levels. Every time they eat, their blood glucose increases rapidly and stays high for the following two to three hours. During that time, excess glucose circulates to all the tissues and organs around the body. The cells lining the blood vessels and those in the eyes and kidneys are extremely vulnerable because they can't control the amount of glucose that enters them. The end result is oxidative stress caused by highly reactive oxygen molecules. These 'free radicals' inflame cells lining arteries, eventually causing swelling, scarring, thickening, hardening and the inability to dilate and contract as needed. In time, the chances of a small blood clot lodging and blocking a narrow artery increases. If it happens in a major vessel of the heart, you have a heart attack on your hands. If it's a minor vessel in the heart, it causes chest pain (angina). If it happens in the brain, it's called a stroke.

But that's not all: high blood glucose levels affect the function of many proteins and enzymes, such that the chances of dying prematurely from any cause are higher. You don't need to be in the diabetic range to be at risk. High glucose and insulin levels fuel the growth of abnormal cells that cause various types of cancer—breast, colon, endometrial and pancreatic—which have all been associated with high blood glucose.

High glucose levels also spell trouble for weight control because insulin will be secreted in an effort to bring glucose down. High insulin in turn causes insulin resistance, causing even higher insulin levels—a vicious cycle. Insulin drives glucose into the 'engines' in each cell, forcing them to burn glucose and pushing fat to the side. In time, fat accumulates all around the body—in the blood (causing high triglycerides), in the liver (causing fatty liver) and in the abdomen (causing the most dangerous form of excess body fat).

Rapid rises and falls in blood glucose are also blamed for increasing appetite. The suddenly low glucose level stimulates the release of stress hormones such as cortisol which stimulate hunger, causing you to think about the next meal. Studies show that slowly digested and absorbed low-GI smart carbs induce greater satiety, delaying the time to the next meal and/or reducing energy intake in comparison to their quickly digested counterparts.

'I have lost approximately 10 kilos . . . and I feel terrific.' – Fil

I am in my early 40s and two years ago, I decided to commit to a regular exercise regime AND a low-GI diet. I have lost approximately 10 kilos in the process and I feel terrific. I can also sense that my body is more appreciative of the way I am treating it than ever before. I had follow-up blood tests about 2 months ago which confirmed that all pre-diabetes triggers (cholesterol, sugar levels, triglycerides, etc.) had fallen well below the acceptable limits which is a fantastic turnaround based on earlier results some 8 months earlier.

Getting both medical and physical confirmation about the benefits of my new lifestyle changes has been such a positive experience and I can only say thank you to the whole GI team on providing me with the information I needed at the right time. I feel very fortunate to have been able to 'reverse' some of the telltale signs associated with men in my age group and look forward to encouraging the rest of my family to embrace this lifestyle as well because the results simply speak for themselves. Bring on the next City to Surf I say!

Week 3 Menu Plan

	BREAKFAST	SNACK	
MONDAY	Natural muesli with low-fat yoghurt and peach slices	Whole-wheat crackers and low-fat sliced cheese	
TUESDAY	Multigrain English muffin melts: top with creamed corn, sliced mushrooms and low-fat mozzarella	2 kiwi fruit or mandarins	
WEDNESDAY	Grainy toast spread with your favourite nut butter, plus a bowl of fresh chopped melon	Fresh carrot and pineapple juice	
THURSDAY	Fruit and nut bar and a skim milk cappuccino	A handful of cherries or other small fruit	
FRIDAY	Egg flip made with low-fat milk, whole egg, vanilla and sugar	An apple	
SATURDAY	Sweetcorn fritters with fried tomato and onion	A bunch of grapes	
SUNDAY	Sautéed mushrooms with parsley and shallots on low-GI toast with a poached egg	A small banana	

LUNCH	SNACK	DINNER
Pasta salad with canned corn, peas, diced red capsicum, grated carrot, chopped tomato and mayonnaise	Small handful of almonds	Pan-fry a lean steak then deglaze pan by adding a little red wine, beef stock and 1 teaspoon Dijon mustard. Simmer for a minute then pour over steaks. Serve with steamed or microwaved new potatoes and broccoli
Flat bread with hummus, tabbouli salad and felafel	Low-fat banana smoothie	Dust boneless fish fillets (e.g. ocean perch) in cornflour. Melt 1 teaspoon margarine in a frypan and add the juice of an orange and a lemon. Add the fish, cover and poach until starting to flake, turning once. Serve with steamed vegetables
Canned tuna with lettuce, tomato, cucumber, feta, olives and balsamic dressing with a grainy roll	A bunch of grapes	Eggplant and Zucchini Pilaf with Lamb (see pages 244–5), plus a low-fat fruit yoghurt
Sweet potato salad: grilled red capsicum with steamed sweet potato and salad greens in balsamic dressing	Grainy toast and chocolate hazelnut spread	Tomato and onion omelette with green salad, plus sliced pineapple and low-fat ice-cream
Cheese, tomato, lettuce, beetroot and grated carrot on a grainy sandwich	Low-fat yoghurt	Chicken and Rice Salad (see page 240)
Stir-fry Asian mixed vegetables with cubed firm tofu and garlic, ginger, soy sauce and honey, stirred through Hokkien noodles	A handful of popcorn and a small orange juice	Rosemary-studded rack of lamb with sweet potato mash, green beans and slow-roasted tomatoes, plus a low-fat chocolate mousse
Salmon frittata with tomato onion salsa, salad greens and a slice of sourdough bread	Fruit with a scoop of low-fat ice-cream	Vegetarian (bean) nachos made with salt-reduced oven-baked corn chips, served with avocado salsa

Week 4

You are four weeks into the Weight-loss Plan now, so it is a good time to re-evaluate your food quantities based on your current weight, using the energy tables on page 45.

Focus on the following goals this week:

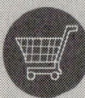

FOOD GOAL

Lowering the GI of your diet with less processed foods.

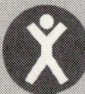

EXERCISE GOAL

Aim to walk at a slightly more brisk, but still comfortable pace (level 4 of the PRE scale), for a total of 20 minutes on five days. *Plus* try to complete each of the two resistance workouts, focusing on the upper and lower body respectively, twice during the week.

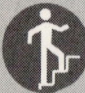

ACTIVITY GOAL

Whenever you are talking on the telephone, stand up, pace the floor and have a stretch.

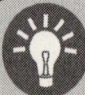

FOOD FOR THOUGHT

How and why foods vary in their GI.

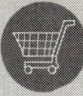

> **FOOD GOAL**
>
> Lowering the GI of your diet with less processed foods.

Porridge, barley, split peas and lentils are remnants from our grandparents' generation that once served us so well. Today we recognise these as some of the lowest GI foods— high in fibre, rich in nutrients, bulky and filling—it is a shame they dwindled in popularity. Once, a hearty bowl of porridge was enough to sustain a person through their morning; now, many people rely on a quick bowl of crispy light flakes. This highly processed alternative is digested so quickly that it spikes blood glucose and insulin levels and leaves you hungry by mid-morning.

This week, consider how many processed foods you rely on and come up with alternatives. Wise ways to lower the GI of your diet include:

- Choose less processed starchy foods—use rolled oats, pearl barley, lentils, split peas and chickpeas. Limit commercial crackers, biscuits and cakes.
- Look for low-GI snacks such as low-fat yoghurts, fresh fruit, dried fruit and nut mix, and low-fat milk.
- Combine high-GI with low-GI foods to produce an intermediate overall GI—lentils plus rice, tabbouli plus bread and potato mixed with sweet potato.
- Add a little acid to your meal—vinaigrette with salad, yoghurt with cereal, lemon juice on vegetables, sourdough bread. All of these contain acids, which slow stomach emptying and lower your blood glucose response to the carbohydrate with which they are eaten.

AIM FOR AT LEAST ONE SMART CARB PER MEAL.

EXERCISE GOAL

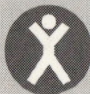

Aim to walk at a slightly more brisk, but still comfortable pace (level 4 of the PRE scale), for a total of 20 minutes on five days. *Plus* try to complete each of the two resistance workouts, focusing on the upper and lower body respectively, twice during the week.

Resistance exercises

We have now split the resistance training into two workouts. The first focuses on the lower body and the second on the upper body. The 'core' abdominals and back are worked in each one as these areas are so important for your posture and strength.

Workout 1	Lower body exercises	'Core' strength abdominals and back
	Squats 2 sets of 10	Three-quarter hover 2 x 20 seconds
	Lunges 10 each leg	
Workout 2	**Upper body exercises**	
	Assisted push-ups 2 sets of 10	Leg extensions 10 each leg
	Standing tricep extensions 2 sets of 10	

NEW EXERCISES

Three-quarter hover

This exercise is fantastic for developing core strength and narrowing your waist. It may feel quite challenging to start with, but you will be amazed at how quickly you improve and reap the rewards of your efforts.

Strengthens and tones: waist

How to do it:

1 Lie face-down on the floor with your toes turned under and prop yourself up on your elbows.

2 Now lift your hips until they are in line with your shoulders and feet—it's important to make sure you don't stick your bottom out but maintain a straight line through the body from shoulder to knee.

3 As you hold the position think of narrowing your waist and breathe normally throughout.

How long: Hold the hover position for 20 seconds, rest for a few moments and then repeat for a further 20 seconds.

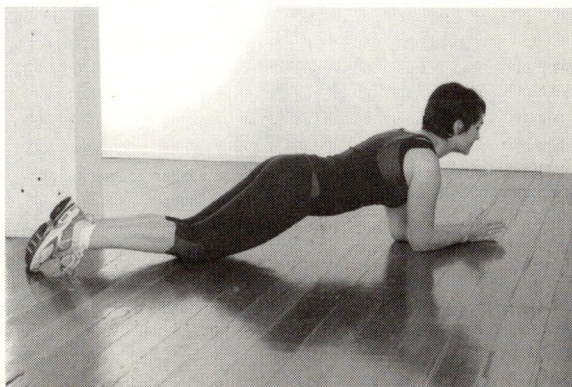

Standing tricep extensions

The back of the upper arms is a common problem area for women in particular—we tend to store body fat here and lack muscle tone. You will need a weight to provide resistance in this exercise. You can buy small hand-held weights at any good sports shop or department store. Alternatively, improvise from your kitchen cupboard: a bag of rice or an unopened can can be used as a good starting weight—anything around the 400-gram mark.

Strengthens and tones: the back of the upper arm

How to do it:

1 Stand tall and hold the weight overhead with both hands (you can also alternate, so one at a time), with your arms straight. Make sure you are standing with good posture and eyes straight ahead, rather than looking up at the weight.

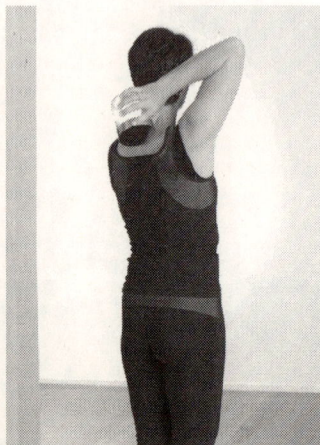

2 Keeping your arms close to your ears, lower the weight behind your head.

3 Keeping the upper arm still, lift the weight back to the top.

How many: 2 sets of 10 with a short rest between sets

Sample diary

Monday	Tuesday	Wednesday	Thursday	Friday	Saturday	Sunday
20 min walk	20 min walk		20 min walk		20 min walk	20 min walk
+ workout 1	+ workout 2		+ workout 1		+ workout 2	
25 mins	25 mins		25 mins		25 mins	20 mins

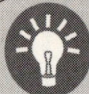

> ### 💡 FOOD FOR THOUGHT
> How and why foods vary in their GI.

From a weight-loss point of view, the longer the process of digestion takes and the more gradual the rise and fall in blood glucose, the better. You don't have to eat all your carbs in low-GI forms. Studies have shown that when a low and a high-GI food are combined in one meal (such as lentils and rice), the overall blood glucose response is intermediate between the two. You can keep both glucose and insulin levels lower over the course of the whole day if you choose at least one low-GI food at each meal.

What determines a food's GI value?

The speed with which carbs reach the bloodstream has little to do with sugar or fibre content. In fact, many sugary foods produce lower blood glucose responses—gram for gram of carbohydrate—than many wholemeal products. By far the most important factor is the physical state of the starch in a food. If the starch granules have swollen and burst, that food will be digested in a flash. On the other hand, if they are still present in their 'native' state as found in the raw food, then the process of digestion will take much longer. Advances in food processing over the past 100 years have had a profound effect on the overall GI values of the carbohydrates we eat.

How do we know if a food is low GI?

The only sure way of knowing the GI value of a food is by measuring it. This means having a group of volunteers eat the food in a controlled setting and comparing their blood glucose levels after the food with their levels after the same carbohydrate load of a standard food, such as glucose. It is a lengthy and labour-intensive procedure, but at least 1500 foods have already been tested and more are being tested all the time in laboratories around the world.

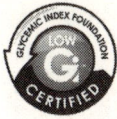

Watch out for this symbol on foods! It is your guarantee that the GI value on the label is correct (it has been tested by an accredited laboratory). This will also assure you that the food makes a nutritious contribution to your diet. Visit the website for more details: **www.gisymbol.com.au**

Factors that influence the GI of a food

Carbohydrate

Remember, only carbohydrate foods have GI values. So any food that is high in carbohydrate has a measurable GI value, but you can't guess what it is without testing it by the standard procedure. If the carbohydrate is predominantly in the form of starch, particularly cooked starch, the food is likely to have a high GI.

Example: cooked flour products such as bread, pancakes and doughnuts

Fat

Fat tends to slow down stomach emptying so high-fat foods often have lower GI values. This doesn't necessarily make high-fat foods good for you.

Example: potato chips, french fries

Protein

If your carbohydrate food is also high in protein, its GI may be lower thanks to slower digestion or a higher insulin response.

Example: Kellogg's® Special K®

Acidity

Just like fat, acid tends to slow down stomach emptying and lowers the GI of carbohydrate foods with which it is eaten. Sometimes the food itself is acidic by nature.

Example: vinaigrette on salad eaten with bread

Soluble fibre

Although you can't see soluble fibre in food, the way it increases the viscosity of your intestinal contents will slow down carbohydrate digestion and lower the GI.

Example: rolled oats

Is it as nature intended?

The less processed the food, the more likely it is to have a low GI. The intact seed coat around wholegrains contributes to their low GI.

Example: legumes

Sugar

Just because a food is sweet, it doesn't make it high GI. The GI depends on the type of sugar and the other sources of carbohydrate in the food. Table sugar or sucrose has an intermediate GI.

'It had been so long since I felt "good" after a meal.' – Amy

I am telling you this 100 per cent true story about my ongoing experience with the low-GI diet. It actually seems a little ridiculous to even call it a 'diet'. It is so easy to follow, and makes so much sense. I laugh every time I think of the time and money I wasted on other diets. I am a nurse, and very serious about researching everything before I try it. Well, I was surprised at the research I did about this low GI thing. It made perfect sense. I have battled, I mean REALLY battled, with digestive problems for about six years. I have had fertility problems, acid reflux, terrible bloating and weight gain throughout the past six long years.

I have been eating only low-GI foods, and very occasionally I will eat a moderate GI food, for about 2 weeks now. I was able to stop taking my Prilosec (which I was totally dependent on) after two days. I stopped taking all my other digestive medications after three days. My bloating ended after day one. I am completely satisfied after a low-GI meal. Not bloated, not tired, not miserable . . . just satisfied. It took me a few days to realise what that actually felt like. It had been so long since I felt 'good' after a meal! I have lost 6 pounds in two weeks. Yep. SIX pounds! I feel GREAT! I have so much more energy than I did before. I look great, and my husband has started on the plan too!

Week 4 Menu Plan

	BREAKFAST	SNACK	
MONDAY	Traditional rolled oat porridge	A handful of peanuts in their shell	
TUESDAY	Half a grapefruit followed by boiled eggs with sourdough toast	An orange	
WEDNESDAY	Natural muesli with sliced apple, low-fat milk and natural yoghurt	A handful of dried apricots	
THURSDAY	Fruit salad with low-fat natural yoghurt and a sprinkle of mixed nuts and seeds	Low-fat flavoured milk	
FRIDAY	Traditional rolled oats topped with fresh or frozen raspberries and low-fat natural yoghurt	Low-fat fruit yoghurt	
SATURDAY	Poached eggs with wilted spinach, grilled tomato and dry-fried mushrooms with a slice of grainy bread	A cup of vegetable soup	
SUNDAY	Heavy fruit toast with low-fat cream cheese and finely sliced apple or pear	A handful of cherries	

LUNCH	SNACK	DINNER
Bowl of minestrone soup with grainy bread dipped in a teaspoon of olive oil	A pear	Grilled lean lamb fillets sliced and served on a sweet potato salad and topped with some tzatziki
Mixed box of sushi with miso soup	Small handful of dried fruit and nut mix	Grilled salmon fillet with mashed sweet potato and steamed broccoli, green beans and carrots
Toasted grainy bread topped with a small can of baked beans and served with a raw tomato	Slice of multigrain toast with a teaspoon of peanut butter	Cover a skinless chicken breast with a basic tomato sauce (ready-made is fine) and bake for 30 minutes. Serve with a steamed corn, wilted spinach and dry-fried mushrooms
Fill a wholemeal pita bread with hummus, tabbouli, lettuce and sliced tomato	Fresh fruit	Chilli con carne made with premium beef mince and kidney beans, serve with steamed Doongara CleverRice, Moolgiri or Basmati rice and a green salad
Steak sandwich—grilled minute steak in multigrain bread with lettuce, beetroot, grated carrot, tomato and mustard	Carrot sticks with hummus dip	Bake a firm white fish fillet in white wine, lemon juice, chopped ginger, garlic and coriander for 20 minutes. Serve with steamed low-GI rice and stir-fried Asian greens in oyster sauce
Lentil soup with grainy bread and low-fat cheese	Strawberries with natural yoghurt and flaked toasted almonds	Grill a chicken breast, slice and serve over a small bowl of pasta in tomato sauce plus a large green salad
Tuna salad with rocket, shallots, baby beets, olives, tomatoes, cucumber, blanched green beans and capsicum, with a little olive oil and balsamic vinegar	Muesli and Honey Slice (see page 264)	Grilled or barbecued pork skewers marinated in spicy sauce. Serve with a large mixed salad and a few baby new potatoes

Week 5

We have already learnt that low-GI foods keep us full for longer and this week we focus on how protein-rich foods can also help. Focus on the following goals this week:

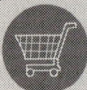

FOOD GOAL
Incorporate a lean protein source in every meal.

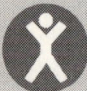

EXERCISE GOAL
Aim to walk at the same pace as last week (level 4 of the PRE scale) for a total of 20 minutes on six days. *Plus* try to complete each of the two resistance workouts, focusing on the upper and lower body respectively, three times during the week.

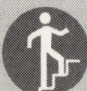

ACTIVITY GOAL
Whenever there is the option of taking the stairs, the lift or an escalator, choose to take the stairs for at least one flight. If you are heading for the 12th floor of a building, for example, take the stairs to the first floor before taking the lift the rest of the way.

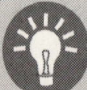

FOOD FOR THOUGHT
The real deal on protein and health.

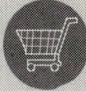

FOOD GOAL

Incorporate a lean protein source in every meal.

Clearly the best foods for weight control would be those that filled you up and stopped you from getting hungry again too quickly. Protein-rich foods tend to be the most satiating, followed by carbohydrate-rich and, in last place, fat-rich foods. In practical terms, this means that by including a protein-rich food in each meal, you can help to satisfy your appetite and delay the return of hunger, seeing you through to the next meal or snack.

While it is unlikely that you have been eating insufficient protein to meet your body's needs, if you have been focusing on reducing your fat intake, you may have inadvertently made it difficult for yourself by omitting the power of protein-rich foods to fill you up. Typical dieters' lunches of a salad sandwich or bowl of vegetable soup may sound like a healthy choice, but on their own these meals are likely to leave you ravenous within a couple of hours of eating them, particularly if the meal included high-GI carbs such as white bread. Add a protein-rich food to the meal, along with a moderate portion of a low-GI carb, and you have a more balanced and filling meal.

For example:

- At breakfast include low-fat milk, yoghurt, eggs, baked beans, lean bacon, smoked salmon, sardines, cottage cheese, ricotta cheese, herrings, nuts or nut butters.
- At light and main meals include lean meat, poultry, fish, reduced-fat cheese, eggs, tofu or legumes (beans or lentils).

EXERCISE GOAL

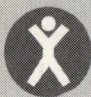

Aim to walk at the same pace as last week (level 4 of the PRE scale) for a total of 20 minutes on six days. *Plus* try to complete each of the two resistance workouts, focusing on the upper and lower body respectively, three times during the week.

Resistance exercises

Workout 1	Lower body exercises	'Core' strength abdominals and back
	Squats 2 sets of 10	Three-quarter hover 2 × 20 seconds
	Lunges 10 each leg	Pointer 10 each side
Workout 2	Upper body exercises	
	Assisted push-ups 2 sets of 10	Leg extensions 10 each leg
	Standing tricep extensions 2 sets of 10	

NEW EXERCISE

Pointer

This is a simple but effective exercise for strengthening the back and bottom muscles, as well as continuing to work on your core abdominal strength.

Strengthens and tones: back, bottom and core abdominals

How to do it:

1 Start on all fours and align your spine by keeping your eyes on the floor just in front of your hands and pulling your navel up towards your spine, without allowing your back to arch. Both your hands and knees should be hip- and shoulder-width apart.

2 Lift your right hand and left leg and extend slowly over a count of four until they are straight and in line with your torso—you are aiming for length rather than height. Hold for 4 seconds before slowly pulling the arm and leg back in close to the torso, then repeat the movement.

3 Repeat with the left arm and right leg.

How many: Repeat 10 extensions on each side.

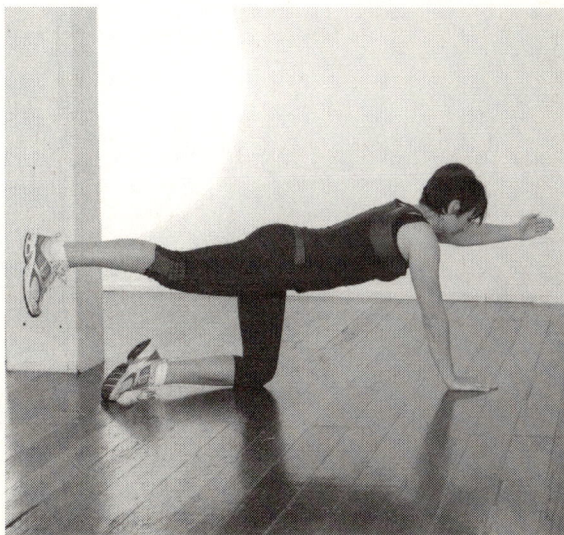

Sample diary

Monday	Tuesday	Wednesday	Thursday	Friday	Saturday	Sunday
20 min walk	20 min walk	20 min walk	20 min walk		20 min walk	20 min walk
+ workout 1	+ workout 2	+ workout 1	+ workout 2		+ workout 1	+ workout 2
30 mins	30 mins	30 mins	30 mins		30 mins	30 mins

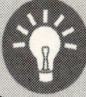

FOOD FOR THOUGHT
The real deal on protein and health.

Adding more protein to your diet makes good sense for weight control. In comparison with carbohydrate and fat, protein makes us feel more satisfied immediately after eating and reduces hunger between meals. In addition, protein increases our metabolic rate for one to three hours after eating. This means we burn more energy by the minute compared with the increase that occurs after eating carbs or fats. Protein foods are also excellent sources of micronutrients, such as iron, zinc, vitamin B12 and omega-3 fats.

Which foods are high in protein?

The highest sources of protein are meats (beef, pork, lamb, chicken), fish and shellfish. As long as these are trimmed of fat and not overlaid with creamy sauces, you can basically eat to suit your appetite. You will find there are natural limits on your appetite for lean protein. Go for the leanest cuts in the supermarket, cut off all the visible (selvage) fat and panfry, grill, bake, stir-fry or barbecue.

Dairy products are not only good sources of protein— the combination of protein and calcium that is unique to dairy foods can aid weight control. The more calcium or dairy foods (it's hard to separate the two) people eat, the lower their weight and fat mass. Calcium is intimately involved in the burning of fat—and that is something we want to encourage! Choose low-fat dairy products including milk, yoghurt and cottage cheese. Go easy on high-fat cheeses such as cheddar, feta, camembert and brie. You don't have to cut them out completely though. It is preferable to have a small serve of these than a giant serve of some reduced-fat version that doesn't taste anywhere near as good.

Nuts are excellent sources of protein and micronutrients but we have to be careful not to overdo them, as they are energy dense—they pack a lot of kilojoules into a small weight. While it is easy to overeat nuts, you don't necessarily have to avoid them. They are high in the good fats. People who eat a small serve of nuts each day have significantly less risk of heart disease. We suggest you have about 30 grams most days. Put a small handful in a small bowl—don't eat straight from the pack.

It is a great shame that eggs have an undeserved bad reputation because of their cholesterol content—in fact they are great sources of protein and several essential vitamins and minerals. We now know that high blood cholesterol results from eating large amounts of saturated fat (rather than cholesterol) in foods. If you select the 'omega-3 enriched' eggs on the market, you are boosting the good fats along with your protein intake.

Can you eat too much protein?

The American Institute of Medicine recommends that no more than 35 per cent of energy in our diets comes from protein. That is 175 grams of pure protein for a person consuming 8500 kilojoules a day. In practice, most people will have no desire to eat beyond that amount.

A high protein intake has been criticised because it might also mean a high intake of saturated fat. That is not true if you stick to lean meat and low-fat dairy products. Concerns about the effect of high protein intake on kidney function are limited to people who already have compromised kidney function: people with diabetes, the very elderly and young infants.

Week 5 Menu Plan

	BREAKFAST	SNACK	LUNCH	
MONDAY	Muesli with fruit and low-fat yoghurt	Grainy cracker and Vegemite®	Toasted cheese and apple sandwich	
TUESDAY	Grainy toast spread with avocado and topped with lean grilled bacon and sliced fresh tomato	An apple	Plain hamburger with lettuce, tomato, beetroot, onion and sauce	
WEDNESDAY	Commercial breakfast drink and a nut bar	Snack pack of peaches	Vegetarian doner kebab with felafel and tabbouli	
THURSDAY	Grainy toast with peanut butter, Yellowbox honey and sliced banana	Low-fat yoghurt	Grainy sandwich with ham and salad	
FRIDAY	Fresh or canned fruit salad with low-fat natural yoghurt and a sprinkle of mixed nuts and seeds	Raisin toast with a light spread of canola margarine	Chickpea salad: mix canned chickpeas, button mushrooms, diced red onion, capsicum, parsley and mint with vinaigrette dressing	
SATURDAY	Baked beans and scrambled egg with low-GI toast	A handful of dried apricots	Bruschetta with tomato topping and a frozen yoghurt ice-cream cone	
SUNDAY	Grilled tomato, egg and grainy toast	A banana	Minestrone soup and a small grainy roll	

SNACK	DINNER
Low-fat chocolate mousse	Tuna pasta with tomato and cucumber salad
Low-fat yoghurt and fresh fruit	Chicken Stuffed with Spinach and Cheese (see page 239) served with sweet potato mash
Snack-size (25–30 g) chocolate bar	Homemade fried rice using Doongara CleverRice
A fresh pear	Spaghetti bolognaise: make your favourite bolognaise sauce with lean minced beef, allowing about 120 g mince per person. Serve with spaghetti (1 cup cooked per person) and a big green side salad tossed in vinaigrette or balsamic dressing
An apple	Panfry boneless fish fillets for 2–3 minutes on each side with a spray of olive oil. Serve with a squeeze of lemon, black pepper and baby new potatoes, steamed broccoli florets, carrot and asparagus spears
An apple	Quick Thai noodle curry: stir-fry some diced trim tofu, sliced onion, red capsicum strips, baby corn, and snowpeas in a large pan. Add 1 tablespoon red curry paste. Prepare Asian noodles according to packet directions and add to vegetables with enough stock to make a sauce. Stir in 1 tablespoon light coconut milk and heat through
Dried fruit and nut mix	Barbecued steak with corn, tomato, mushrooms and salad

Week 6

This week is all about changing your thinking on fats and seeing the good as well as the bad. Focus on the following goals this week:

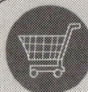

FOOD GOAL

Break out of the 'low fat' dieting mentality.

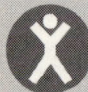

EXERCISE GOAL

Aim to walk at the same pace as last week (level 4 of the PRE scale) for a total of 20 minutes on six days. *Plus* try to complete each of the two resistance workouts, focusing on the upper and lower body respectively, three times during the week.

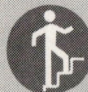

ACTIVITY GOAL

For every hour that you spend sitting down, get up and do something more active for five minutes—have a quick stretch, walk to the printer, hang out the washing or complete some other household or office chore.

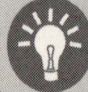

FOOD FOR THOUGHT

The fats of the matter.

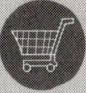

FOOD GOAL

Break out of the 'low fat' dieting mentality.

Your food goal this week involves looking at the fats in your diet—not to discard them, but to ensure that you are eating the right balance of good and bad fats. By allowing yourself to incorporate healthy fats you will enjoy your meals more (fat tastes good) and gain the long-term benefits of fat-soluble vitamins and anti-oxidants. The following are the guidelines we recommend.

Eat less saturated fat

Reducing your total fat intake will lower the energy density of your diet and help you lose weight, but it is important to focus on specifically reducing the saturated fats as your highest priority. Saturated fats should constitute less than 10 per cent of total kilojoules for the day. For a person eating 6400 kilojoules this means eating less than 16 grams of saturated fat per day. (See table on page 113.)

Boost your omega-3 intake

These unique fats found in seafood can reduce inflammation in the body, iron out irregularities in heart beat, reduce blood fat levels and might play a valuable role in treating depression and Alzheimer's disease. Modern Western diets almost certainly do not provide enough of the polyunsaturated omega-3 fats. Around 650 milligrams of omega-3 fats are considered an adequate daily intake for adults. The following foods contain approximately 650 milligrams of omega-3 fats:

- 40 g canned sardines
- 30 g canned mackerel
- 40 g smoked salmon
- 30 g canned red salmon
- 50 g canned pink salmon
- 110 g fresh Atlantic salmon
- 180 g canned tuna
- 4 omega-3 eggs

Replace bad fats with good fats

Replacing saturated fats with monounsaturated fats will lower your bad cholesterol and increase your good cholesterol.

- Substitute butter with canola margarines and spreads.
- Use liquid oils (or oil-based sprays) for frying, including canola and olive oils.
- Cold-pressed olive oil contains anti-oxidants that are not found in refined oils.
- Check for the presence of these oils (such as canola or olive) in commercially fried and 'oven-bake' products (if you use them), in preference to animal fats and unspecified vegetable oils.
- Use low-fat milk (or soy substitute) in place of full-cream milk.
- Eat a handful of nuts as an alternative to potato chips and other commercial packet snacks.

Grams of saturated fat found in everyday servings of common foods

Chicken drumstick, 1 including skin	4 g
Cream cheese, 1 tablespoon	4 g
Sausage, 1 thin	4 g
Lamb loin chop (not trimmed), 1 grilled	4 g
Milk chocolate, 4 squares, 30 g	5 g
Sour cream, 1 tablespoon	5 g
Cream, 1 tablespoon	6 g
Milk, full fat, 1 cup	6 g
Rich chocolate cake, iced and filled, 1 piece, 100 g	6 g
Salami, 2 thin slices	6 g
Pizza, supreme, 2 slices	6 g
Cheddar cheese, 40 g	7 g
Chips, 50 g packet	7 g
Hamburger, 1 average	7 g
Shortbread, 3 biscuits	7 g
Butter, 1 tablespoon	10 g
Croissant, 1	10 g
Doughnut, 1 cinnamon and sugar	10 g
Meat pie, 1	10 g
Cheesecake, 1 large slice, 120 g	12 g
Sausage roll, 1 small	17 g
Coconut cream, 140 g can	25 g
Fried chicken takeaway meal, average	25 g

EXERCISE GOAL

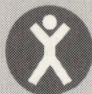

Aim to walk at the same pace as last week (level 4 of the PRE scale) for a total of 20 minutes on six days. *Plus* try to complete each of the two resistance workouts, focusing on the upper and lower body respectively, three times during the week.

Resistance exercises

This week we make the resistance exercises you have already learnt a little harder by omitting the rest between sets.

Workout 1	Lower body exercises	'Core' strength abdominals and back
	Squats 1 set of 20	Three-quarter hover 2 × 30 seconds
	Lunges 10 each leg	Pointer 10 each side
Workout 2	**Upper body exercises**	
	Assisted push-ups 1 set of 20	Leg extensions 10 each leg
	Standing tricep extensions 1 set of 20	Ab curl 1 set of 20

NEW EXERCISE

Ab curl

Now that we have started to strengthen the deep abdominal muscles involved in posture and support of the lower back, we can add an exercise for the outer muscles. A basic ab curl works the sixpack—these are the ab muscles that you use to sit up from lying down or to curl the torso forward. It is crucial to continue working the core muscles as well so that you strengthen and tone from the inside out. The old-fashioned ab curl you may remember from school days (where you hooked your feet under a bar and sat up all the way) is not a good idea—this simply pulls into play your hip flexor muscles instead of making the abs do all the work.

Note: Without great care this exercise can strain the back and neck.

Strengthens and tones: the sixpack abs

How to do it:
1 Lie on the floor with your knees bent and your feet flat on the floor.
2 Lightly place your fingertips behind your ears and keep your elbows pointing to the side to avoid pulling on your head and neck.
3 Pull in your navel and curl your torso up about 45 degrees, then return to the floor.

Remember:
- Keep the small of the back in contact with the floor.
- Imagine you are holding an orange under your chin to maintain a space between your chin and chest.
- Keep your eyes focused diagonally over your knees rather than looking straight up at the ceiling—a good place to look is where the ceiling meets the wall.

How many: 20 curls

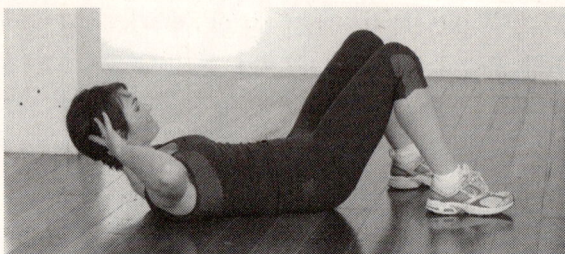

Sample diary

Monday	Tuesday	Wednesday	Thursday	Friday	Saturday	Sunday
20 min walk	20 min walk	20 min walk	20 min walk		20 min walk	20 min walk
+ workout 1	+ workout 2	+ workout 1	+ workout 2		+ workout 1	+ workout 2
30 mins	30 mins	30 mins	30 mins		30 mins	30 mins

Congratulations, you are halfway through the 12-week Weight-loss Plan

Remember, the low-GI diet is not a fad diet. It is a serious diet and exercise program aimed at reducing body fat and *keeping it off for life*. Completing the plan is the first step to better health and weight loss—and you are halfway there. Congratulations. Remember it is a blueprint for healthy eating for the rest of your life. The 12-week Weight-loss Plan is followed by step two, 'Doing it for Life', which gives you the whole weight-loss *tool kit*—an assortment of strategies and tips to make lifestyle change easier, incorporating food, exercise and behavioural change. The GI is just one of these tools but, nonetheless, an important one that makes a world of difference to your chances of successful long-term weight control.

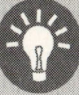

> ### 💡 FOOD FOR THOUGHT
> The fats of the matter.

To most people, 'low fat' is still synonymous with 'healthy' and 'weight loss'. Unfortunately, it is not that simple. Once upon a time, when fruit, vegetables and wholegrains were the staples of a low-fat diet this might have been true. But it is no longer so—indeed, the typical low-fat diet may be distinctly unhealthy and one of the reasons behind our expanding waistlines.

In the 1990s, the experts told us to eat low-fat diets because they were concerned about two things. First, they believed saturated fat increased the risk of heart disease, and second, that fatty foods were too easily overeaten because they were energy dense. Those concerns are still valid today—the experts haven't changed their minds again. But the solution to the problem—eating a low-fat diet—has not been a successful strategy. While we have cut down on total fat, we haven't cut down on saturated fat, and the food industry (with the best of intentions) gave us a myriad of low-fat foods that were just as energy dense as their full fat counterparts. So during the 1990s, the era of '99 per cent fat free', the prevalence of obesity soared and with it heart disease and diabetes.

As a result of these unexpected events, the heart foundations and health organisations around the world went back to the drawing board and remodelled their dietary advice, as follows:

1 The *type* of fat is more important for health than the total amount.

2 The energy density of a food (kilojoules per 100 grams) is more important to weight control than the fat content.

Furthermore, most of us need to eat more of certain kinds of fat for optimal health (yes, you read it right). These include the omega-3 fats found in fish and seafood, walnuts and canola-based products. Eating these and more monounsaturated fats such as those in olive oil and canola oil has been shown to reduce the risk of heart attack significantly. Indeed, one of the most important diet studies ever carried out, the Lyon Heart Study, showed that a diet with more fish, fruit, vegetables and good fats was twice as effective in reducing cardiovascular 'events' as the low-fat diet recommended by the American Heart Association. In fact, it is a whole lot better than most of the expensive drugs used to reduce the risk of heart attack.

There is another excellent reason why you should aim to increase these monounsaturated fats at the expense of the saturated ones. While all fats have the same number of kilojoules per gram, they may not all have the same effect on your weight. For reasons that are not yet clear, a high-fat diet based on fish oil or olive oil is much less likely to expand the waistline. Research is also showing that people who eat diets rich in the omega-3 fats are less likely to suffer rheumatoid arthritis, psoriasis, ulcerative colitis, depression (and other mental illness), and possibly some cancers. We recommend that you eat the food fats in the form of food rather than pills or just oils. In the whole food, you get the whole package that nature provided.

Where do you find the good oils?

- Fish such as salmon, tuna, herrings and sardines— canned or fresh
- Shellfish
- Walnuts, almonds and cashews—best unsalted
- Avocado—spread it on as an alternative to margarine or butter
- Spinach, bok choy, leafy green salads
- Olives—spread as a tapenade or add whole to almost anything—pasta sauces, couscous or salads
- Muesli—mix sunflower seeds and pumpkin seeds with ground almonds or hazelnuts
- Linseed (flaxseed) is a great source of omega-3 fats; a good way to eat it is in soy and linseed bread.

A low-fat diet is not necessarily the best diet for weight loss or overall health.

'Fat free' and 'reduced fat' on the label is not a licence to eat more.

Eating less saturated fat and more monounsaturated and omega-3 fats is the best option for long-term health.

Week 6 Menu Plan

	BREAKFAST	SNACK	
MONDAY	Orange and grapefruit segments with prunes and a low-fat honey-flavoured yoghurt, sprinkled with toasted flaked almonds	Raisin toast	
TUESDAY	Soy and linseed toast with margarine and a boiled egg, plus a low-fat milky coffee	A banana	
WEDNESDAY	Muesli with sliced pear and low-fat milk, sprinkled with chopped almonds or hazelnuts	Small vegetable juice, grainy crackers	
THURSDAY	Banana smoothie made with an omega-3 egg	Hot chocolate with low-fat milk	
FRIDAY	Toasted cheese and tomato sandwich and an apple	Low-fat yoghurt	
SATURDAY	High-fibre, low GI cereal with low-fat milk and canned peach slices	Dried fruit biscuits	
SUNDAY	Egg, lean bacon, tomato, mushrooms and grainy toast with grapefruit juice	An apple	

LUNCH	SNACK	DINNER
Miso soup with sushi rolls	An apple	Stir-fried beef with garlic, onion, capsicum, carrot, zucchini and snowpeas dressed with sweet chilli sauce and served with Doongara CleverRice
Chicken and coleslaw on a mixed grain roll with fresh or canned fruit salad	Low-fat milk with Milo®	Spread a round of pita bread with pesto or tomato paste. Top with sliced tomato, mushrooms, roasted capsicum, black olives, chopped spring onions and a sprinkle of grated parmesan cheese. Heat through in a hot oven
Salmon and lettuce sandwich on grainy bread	2 kiwi fruit	Beef stroganoff with mushrooms (substitute light sour cream for sour cream) with fettuccine pasta, steamed broccoli and cauliflower
Lean ham, pineapple and grated light cheese on a toasted, mixed grain muffin	An orange	Commercial oven-bake fish and potato wedges with carrot and zucchini julienne alongside
Steak sandwich made on grainy bread with salad	A banana	Thai-style Tofu and Noodle Soup (see page 235)
Minestrone soup and a crusty white roll	An apple	Thinly slice and pan-fry pork loin steak. Toss with baby spinach, sliced red onion and steamed new potatoes (halved or quartered)
Macaroni cheese made with light milk and reduced-fat cheese. Throw in a bag of frozen mixed vegetables with the macaroni	Snack-size chocolate bar (25–30 g)	Roast leg of lamb with a small roast potato, roast sweet potato, pumpkin, steamed beans and peas, served with mint sauce

Week 7

This week, focus on these goals:

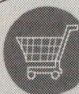

FOOD GOAL

Think about what you are drinking.

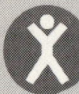

EXERCISE GOAL

Aim to walk at the same pace as last week (level 4 of our PRE scale), but for a total of 25 minutes on six days. *Plus* try to complete each of the two resistance workouts, focusing on the upper and lower body respectively, three times during the week.

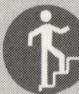

ACTIVITY GOAL

Watch no more than two hours of television on any day and choose one day where you will not watch television at all.

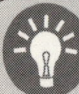

FOOD FOR THOUGHT

Wholegrains—the whole story.

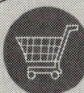

> ### FOOD GOAL
> Think about what you are drinking.

Did you realise that it is a good idea to drink more when you are losing weight? One reason is that a large part of our fluid intake comes from food, so if we are eating less food, we are also taking in less fluid. Additional fluid is also helpful for removing extra toxins which can be released during weight loss. What you choose to drink, however, can have a major impact on your success with weight loss.

Many things we drink would be better thought of as food due to the kilojoules they contain. Fruit juice might sound like a healthy option but ordering a glass of orange juice in a cafe can be the equivalent of the energy (kilojoules) from ten oranges; a large soft drink can provide as many as 15 teaspoons of sugar in a single serve; while a takeaway coffee can contain as much as 10 grams of fat if made with full cream milk. It is not hard to see how the calories can stack up without filling you up.

Of all the things we drink, however, alcohol could be thought of as the most fattening—not because of its kilojoule content, but because it has priority as a fuel over all other nutrients. So basically, as long as there is alcohol in your system, anything else is surplus until the alcohol kilojoules are used up. Looking at it another way, just one can of beer replaces all the calories burnt by 20 minutes of brisk walking.

Your best option for extra fluid is water. Soda water, low-sodium mineral water, herbal teas and decaffeinated drinks are other options. Diet soft drinks are okay—certainly they contain almost no kilojoules, but they are highly acidic (which can soften the enamel of your teeth). Plus, be aware of the caffeine content in these types of drinks, which can be considerable.

When you are trying to lose weight, it is best to think of alcohol as an indulgence. It may be enjoyable but it doesn't provide any essential nutrients and is high in kilojoules. Limit your intake as much as you can. Even when you get to the weight maintenance stage, an average daily limit of no more than two standard drinks for men and one standard drink for women is recommended.

A standard drink is:

- 100 ml wine
- A middy (285 ml) of full strength beer or a schooner of light (410 ml)
- 30 ml spirits
- 60 ml fortified wine (sherry, port, etc.)

Did you know?

Your body reacts differently to fluids compared to food. There is evidence that sugar in liquid form (such as soft drinks and fruit juices) may sneak past the brain's appetite centre. When we chew, signals are sent to the brain that food is on its way and our appetite begins to be altered before the food even hits our stomach. When we drink, however, these signals don't occur and the same level of satiety is not reached, making it easy for us to overconsume.

EXERCISE GOAL

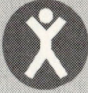

Aim to walk at the same pace as last week (level 4 of our PRE scale), but for a total of 25 minutes on six days. *Plus* try to complete each of the two resistance workouts, focusing on the upper and lower body respectively, three times during the week.

Resistance exercises

Workout 1	Lower body exercises	'Core' strength abdominals and back
	Squats 1 set of 20	Three-quarter hover 2 × 30 seconds
	Lunges 10 each leg	Pointer 10 each side
Workout 2	**Upper body exercises**	
	Assisted push-ups 1 set of 20	Leg extensions 10 each leg
	Standing tricep extensions 1 set of 20	Ab curl 1 set of 20
	Bicep curl 1 set of 20	

NEW EXERCISE

Bicep curl

When working one muscle or group of muscles we should always try to work the opposing muscle(s) to the same extent. This maintains an equilibrium of strength and flexibility across joints and is crucial in achieving good posture and avoiding injuries. We learnt to work the back of the arm last week, therefore this week we need to add an exercise for the front of the arm. A bicep curl is the most effective and simple way to do this.

Strengthens and tones: front of the arm

How to do it:

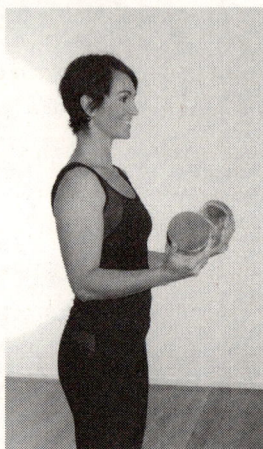

1 Hold your hand weights (or cans) by your sides with your palms facing forward.

2 Maintain good posture through your body, keeping your torso strong and upright throughout.

3 Curl the weights up towards your shoulders, keeping your elbows close to your ribcage, and slowly return to the start position.

How many: Complete 20 curls.

Sample diary

Monday	Tuesday	Wednesday	Thursday	Friday	Saturday	Sunday
25 min walk	25 min walk	25 min walk	25 min walk		25 min walk	25 min walk
+ workout 1	+ workout 2	+ workout 1	+ workout 2		+ workout 1	+ workout 2
35 mins	35 mins	35 mins	35 mins		35 mins	35 mins

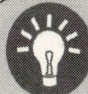

FOOD FOR THOUGHT

Wholegrains—the whole story.

While there is plenty of evidence that wholegrains and cereal fibre are good for you, there are plenty of nutritious foods that are relatively low in fibre and yet full of micronutrients (such as oranges, dairy products, fish and lean meat). In our experience, only a small minority of people is willing to eat cereal products in their true 'native state'. For many people, unrefined foods, such as brown bread, brown rice and brown pasta, are not to their liking.

Humans did not eat large amounts of any cereal grain until the advent of agriculture, a recent event on the evolutionary clock. But once farming became established, we found increasingly ingenious ways of removing the 'brown bits' and making cereal products ever more palatable—probably too palatable for our own good!

Having said this, the benefits of eating more fibre—especially if you are battling the bulge—are obvious. In one study of nearly 3000 young adults, those who ate more fibre (about 25 grams a day) gained much less weight over the years than those who ate the least (less than 10 grams a day). What's more, their fibre intake was a better predictor of the amount of weight gain than their fat intake (the usual suspect). Why? Lots of reasons: high-fibre foods take longer to eat, they are heavier and bulkier, fill you up sooner and leave you feeling more satiated (think of grainy bread versus white bread). Another reason is that eating more wholegrains and fibre has been shown to improve insulin sensitivity and lower insulin levels. That means greater use of fat as a source of fuel—good news if you are trying to lose weight.

There are plenty of other reasons to encourage you to eat more wholegrains if you enjoy them. Higher fibre intake—especially from cereals—has been linked to lower risk of cancer of the large bowel, breast, stomach and mouth. What is the connection? New research shows that high insulin levels increase the multiplication of mutated cells, producing uncontrolled growth of tumours and cancers. Plus, another function of fibre is to bind carcinogenic substances and help sweep them out of the system.

Much of the goodness in grains is found just beneath the bran layer and is usually lost along with the fibre when grains are milled. Vitamins, minerals, anti-oxidants and other protective substances in wholegrains—many of which are not present in nutritional supplements—are also lost. However, some wheats are better than others—when hard wheats, such as durum wheat, are milled into flour or semolina (to make pasta), it is easier to separate the bran, and the final product contains higher quantities of micronutrients.

Our take-home message is to reduce your intake of highly processed and refined cereal products that produce glycemic spikes and leave you craving more. The most obvious examples are soft white bread and low-fat snacks and crackers but also include some foods that are high in fibre—modern wholemeal breads (where you can't see the grain) and brown rice are often quickly digested and absorbed. We recommend you swap some of these high-GI carbohydrates for smart carbs that are slowly digested and absorbed, irrespective of their fibre content. Pasta, noodles, low-GI rices and sourdough bread are good examples of low-GI foods that everyone enjoys. While their fibre content may be low, some of the starch is resistant to digestion and aids large bowel health in the same way that fibre does. If you enjoy the high-fibre version, that's an added bonus!

If a food's label shows at least 3 grams of fibre per serving, consider it a good source. Experts recommend 30 grams of fibre a day. Increase your fibre intake slowly so your bowel flora has time to adapt.

Low-GI sources of fibre (grams per serve)	
Grain bread (lots of whole kernels visible), 1 slice	2
Porridge, 1 cup, cooked	2
Apple, 1 medium, including skin	3
Barley, ½ cup, cooked	3
Corn kernels, 100 g, canned	3
Lentils, ½ cup, cooked	3
Prunes, 5	3
Sweet potato, 120 g, boiled	3
Popcorn, 2 cups, popped	4
Pumpernickel bread, 50 g slice	4
Dried apricots, 6 halves	5
Guardian®, 1 cup	5
Peas, ½ cup, cooked	5
All-Bran®, ½ cup	10
Chickpeas, ½ cup, cooked	10

Week 7 Menu Plan

	BREAKFAST	SNACK	LUNCH	
MONDAY	Grainy bread spread with fresh ricotta and blackberry conserve	A banana	Pasta salad with lean ham, corn kernels, capsicum, shallots and mayonnaise with lettuce	
TUESDAY	Breakfast on the Go (see page 222)	Skim milk latte	Asian seafood combination with vegetables and boiled noodles	
WEDNESDAY	Low-GI, high-fibre breakfast cereal with low-fat milk and sliced banana	Mandarins	Chicken, avocado and salad on grainy bread	
THURSDAY	Low-fat toasted muesli with yoghurt and canned fruit	An apple	Grainy crackers with hummus, sliced tomato, celery and sardines	
FRIDAY	Fruit loaf spread with light cream cheese and topped with sliced apple and a sprinkle of cinnamon	Dried pear halves	Pumpkin soup with grainy toasted croutons and low-fat yoghurt garnish	
SATURDAY	Mushroom, cheese and spinach omelette with grainy toast and a glass of fruit juice	An apple	Steak sandwich: grilled minute steak in multigrain bread with lettuce, beetroot, grated carrot, tomato and mustard	
SUNDAY	Chopped banana stirred into porridge, topped with a drizzle of honey and low-fat milk	Oatmeal biscuits	Sardines or smoked trout, sourdough bread and fresh green salad with lemon and vinegar	

SNACK	DINNER
Low-fat yoghurt	Stir-fry lean beef with grated ginger and crushed garlic. Add snowpeas, broccoli florets, chopped spring onion, Chinese cabbage slices and a little finely chopped chilli. Combine soy and hoisin sauces with honey, toss and serve with Doongara CleverRice
Canned peaches	Panfried chicken breast with mushroom sauce (use light evaporated milk in place of cream), canned butter beans, carrots and green beans
Low-fat fruit yoghurt	Boil a packet of spinach and cheese (or your favourite filling) tortellini according to packet directions. Heat some bottled tomato sauce and serve this on top of the tortellini with a sprinkle of parmesan cheese. Serve with a large salad and vinaigrette
Carrot sticks with hummus	Mediterranean roast vegetables with trimmed lamb cutlets
Orange and Passionfruit Mousse (see page 269)	Mexican bean tacos: fill warm taco shells with 2–3 tablespoons Mexi-beans and top with shredded lettuce, grated reduced-fat cheese and 1–2 teaspoons light sour cream
A banana	Sweet potato wedges (page 250) with oven-baked fish. Wrap fish fillets or cutlets (one per person) in individual foil parcels with a slice of lemon and a twist of freshly ground black pepper, and bake in the oven at 180°C for 10–15 minutes
Baked banana with passionfruit	Ham and Vegetable Bake (see page 229) and salad

Week 8

Many of us assign foods to a 'good' or 'bad' category and inevitably it is the foods we see as treat foods that we see as 'bad'. Yet by allowing yourself to indulge in whatever food/drink you really enjoy, you can diminish the uncontrollable desire to overeat these foods and they become a normal part of eating. Focus on the following goals this week:

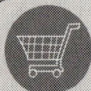

FOOD GOAL
Include an indulgence occasionally.

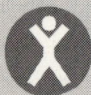

EXERCISE GOAL
Aim to walk for a total of 25 minutes on six days but increase your pace to a brisk walk (of around level 5 of the PRE scale) for the middle 15 minutes. *Plus* try to complete each of the resistance workouts, focusing on the upper and lower body respectively, three times during the week.

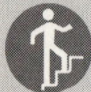

ACTIVITY GOAL
Go shopping on foot and carry your bags home—a fantastic total body workout! (If you have to drive to the nearest shopping centre, park the car in the furthest parking spot and walk the rest of the way.)

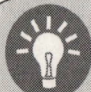

FOOD FOR THOUGHT
Allow yourself something sweet!

> ### FOOD GOAL
> Include an indulgence occasionally.

Have you ever finished your main course and found yourself hankering for a little of something sweet? Do you prefer your tea and coffee with the taste of real sugar? Perhaps you feel that a sweet fix helps you work through the afternoon. Maybe you really enjoy coffee and cake with a good friend once a week. Bad habits? We don't think so.

Just because you have decided to change your eating habits doesn't mean you can't indulge once a week. Imagine yourself at a meeting and suddenly a chocolate mud cake is being offered around. It is okay to enjoy a piece of cake with everyone else, but make the decision to eat—or not eat—an active one. Do you automatically accept a piece of cake (even though you're not hungry) and eat it during the meeting, barely tasting it (passively indulging), or do you consider the look of the cake and how hungry you are and decide it could be a nice change for morning tea (active decision making)? Your thinking and actions in the second instance are more positive than in the first instance, which means you are less likely to feel guilty about indulging.

This week, we want you to look at the feelings you may have about eating certain foods. The aim is for you to make active, guilt-free choices about the foods you eat, confident in the knowledge that you can eat your favourite foods, and still work towards your goals. This is also a good time to revise your basic daily food quantities to be sure your background diet is sound. (See page 45.)

And in case you haven't done so for a while, this week, choose an indulgence that you fancy and go ahead and enjoy it!

Indulgences to savour:

3 jam tartlets

½ slice of cake

2 cream biscuits

40 g of your favourite cheese

1 snack-size (25 g) chocolate bar

2 glasses (200 ml) wine

1 can regular soft drink

2 tablespoons cream

½ small serve French fries

375 ml beer

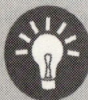

In the era of digital cameras, it is easy to take a weekly shot of your body (full length) side on. Take it in the same place each week (such as inside a door frame) so you can easily see your weekly progress.

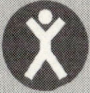

> **EXERCISE GOAL**
>
> Aim to walk for a total of 25 minutes on six days but increase your pace to a brisk walk (of around level 5 of the PRE scale) for the middle 15 minutes. *Plus* try to complete each of the resistance workouts, focusing on the upper and lower body respectively, three times during the week.

Resistance exercises

Workout 1	Lower body exercises	'Core' strength abdominals and back
	Squats 1 set of 20	Full hover 2 × 30 seconds
	Lunges 10 each leg	Pointer 10 each side
	Power lunge 20 alternate legs	
Workout 2	**Upper body exercises**	
	Assisted push-ups 1 set of 20	Leg extensions 10 each leg
	Standing tricep extensions 1 set of 20	Ab curl 1 set of 20
	Bicep curl 1 set of 20	

NEW EXERCISES

Power lunges

This is a more advanced version of the lunge you have already learnt. By adding some movement you recruit all the smaller stabiliser muscles of the legs, the postural muscles have to work hard and you increase the load the major muscles of the legs and bottom have to move. This is a fantastic exercise for toning and strengthening the lower body.

Strengthens and tones: legs and bottom

How to do it:

1 Start with your feet hip-width apart and your arms by your side. Keep your eyes looking straight ahead rather than down at the floor to help you maintain good posture.

2 Take a long step forward with one leg and sink into your lunge, similarly to your usual lunge move, but then push yourself back to standing by driving into your front heel.

3 As you complete the power lunge allow your arms to swing naturally by your sides to help with balance. Repeat on the other leg.

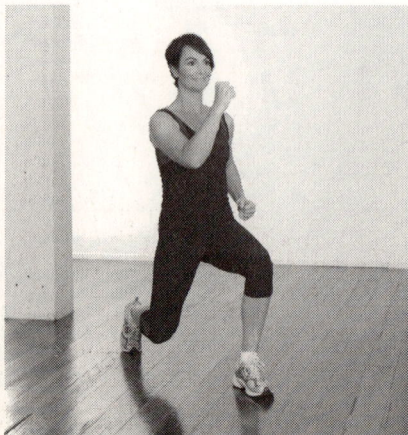

Remember: Keep your chest proud and upper body upright throughout so that all the work is in the legs and bottom muscles.

How many: 20, using alternate legs

Full hover

This is a more advanced level of the three-quarter hover you have already learnt.

Strengthens and tones: core abdominals—improves your posture and narrows your waist

How to do it:

1 Start in your three-quarter hover position (see page 91) and then lift your knees, straightening your legs until your body is in alignment from heel to shoulder.
2 Check that your bottom is not sticking up and that you are not allowing your lower back to sag—pull your navel in towards your spine.
3 Straighten up and keep your hips in line with your body.

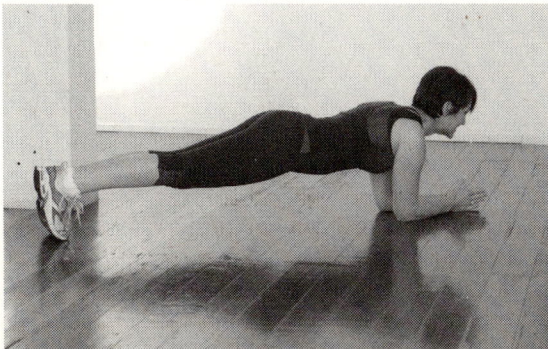

Remember: Breathe normally while you maintain the position—it is very easy to hold your breath without realising.

How long: Hold for 2 sets of 30 seconds with a short rest in between.

Sample diary

Monday	Tuesday	Wednesday	Thursday	Friday	Saturday	Sunday
25 min walk	25 min walk	25 min walk	25 min walk		25 min walk	25 min walk
+ workout 1	+ workout 2	+ workout 1	+ workout 2		+ workout 1	+ workout 2
35 mins	35 mins	35 mins	35 mins		35 mins	35 mins

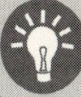

> ### FOOD FOR THOUGHT
> Allow yourself something sweet!

Most people mistakenly believe that sugar is the first thing that ought to go when they are 'on a diet'—it is just 'empty calories' and is probably responsible for one's current state of overweight. We have a prudish notion that if something tastes good, it must be bad for us. However, yearning for something sweet is instinctual and hard to ignore, especially when you are actively losing weight. In our evolutionary past, honey was a significant part of hunter–gatherer diets and a lot more concentrated as a source of sugar than most of the sugary foods we eat today.

In fact, sugar is not specifically implicated in making us fat. In the Baltimore Ageing Study, for example, the best predictor of weight gain over time was a diet characterised by a lot of bread (most varieties being high GI). Those who ate a lot of sweets gained very little— about the same as those who adhered to the principles of healthy eating (lots of fruit, vegetables, wholegrains and lean protein).

It is obvious, too, that the vast array of sugar-free and 'no added sugar' foods on supermarket shelves has not solved the problem of overweight. In fact, it could be said that they have exacerbated the problem by encouraging people to think that using a sugar substitute is all it takes to cut kilojoules and control weight. If only!

Here is a word of caution, however. For example, if you give people 500 extra kilojoules as solid food, they compensate by consuming fewer kilojoules during the rest of the day. But if you feed them 500 kilojoules in a soft drink, juice or other clear liquid, they don't reduce their intake at all. All 500 kilojoules are surplus and may head straight for your hips or waist. Indeed, in a recent study, the children who became overweight were greater consumers of soft drinks and fruit juices.

With a low-GI diet we encourage you to enjoy refined sugar in moderation—that's about 40 to 50 grams a day—an amount that most people consume without thinking about it. Include sweetened foods that pack nutrients, not just kilojoules—dairy foods, breakfast cereals, porridge with brown sugar or jam on grainy toast. Even the World Health Organisation says, '*a moderate intake of sugar-rich foods can provide for a palatable and nutritious diet*'. We want you to cut the guilt trip and allow yourself the pleasure of sweetness. To guide you, let's take a quick look at the sugar content of some common foods.

Refined sugar content of various foods

1 shortbread biscuit	3 g
1 cream filled biscuit	5 g
1 boiled lolly	5 g
1 cup sweetened fruit juice	5 g
1 rounded teaspoon sugar	6 g
1 cinnamon and sugar doughnut	7 g
1 piece plain cake	7 g
1 tablespoon jam	8 g
1 muesli bar (average)	8 g
1 piece chocolate cake	11 g
30 ml undiluted cordial	18 g
5 squares chocolate	20 g
1 tablespoon honey	20 g
1 chocolate bar (average)	35 g
375 ml can soft drink (average)	45 g

Week 8 Menu Plan

	BREAKFAST	SNACK
MONDAY	High-fibre fruit smoothie: blend low-fat milk, natural yoghurt, a banana, a handful of berries and 1 tablespoon psyllium husks	A small handful of raw almonds
TUESDAY	Baked beans on grainy toast followed by an orange	An apple and a wedge of reduced-fat cheddar
WEDNESDAY	Grilled lean bacon and tomato sandwich on sourdough bread	A handful of red grapes
THURSDAY	Traditional porridge served with low-fat milk and a dollop of raspberry jam	Hot chocolate with low-fat milk
FRIDAY	Homemade muesli (blend rolled oats, mixture of dried fruit, nuts and seeds) with low-fat milk and a few sliced strawberries	Low-fat fruit yoghurt
SATURDAY	Egg and bacon with toast, tomato and mushroom	An apple
SUNDAY	Omelette filled with spinach and mushrooms served with toasted sourdough bread	Skim milk latte with a small cake

LUNCH	SNACK	DINNER
Ham sandwich on grainy bread. Lean ham and lots of salad vegies—lettuce, tomato, beetroot, grated carrot and sprouts. Flavour with mustard or chutney	A piece of fruit	Spaghetti bolognaise made with premium beef mince— serve with a large mixed salad, a shaving of parmesan and a small glass of red wine
Tortilla wrap filled with chicken, lettuce, tomato, cucumber and salsa	A small (40 g) chocolate bar	Herbed Fish Parcels with Sweet Potato Wedges and Coleslaw (see page 250)
Tomato and barley soup with grainy bread and low-fat cheese	Skim milk hot chocolate	Chicken and cashew nut stir-fry with capsicum, mushrooms, onion, ginger, garlic, chilli, Asian greens and 1 teaspoon honey. Serve with noodles
Smoked mackerel fillet with a large mixed salad and a slice of sourdough bread, plus a piece of fresh fruit	Your favourite ice-cream	Grilled lean beef steak with a steamed ear of corn and a large mixed salad dressed with a little olive oil and vinegar dressing
Roast beef sandwich on grainy bread with salad vegetables and mustard	Peaches and cream	Salad Niçoise with lettuce, blanched green beans, boiled new potatoes, hard-boiled egg, olives, spring onions, baby gherkins, anchovies and plum tomatoes. Top with fresh or canned tuna and drizzle with olive oil and lemon juice dressing
Mixed bean salad with rocket and a slice of grainy bread	A handful of red grapes	Seafood fettuccine in a tomato-based sauce and a green salad
Barbecued Lamb with Lentil Salad and Lemon Yoghurt Dressing (see page 246)	Fruit salad with natural yoghurt	Quick pita bread pizza: top a pita bread with tomato paste, chopped zucchini, capsicum, tomato and mixed herbs, sprinkle with reduced-fat mozzarella and bake for 20 minutes in a hot oven. Serve with a green salad

Week 9

After two months of changing your eating and exercise habits step by step, you should be feeling and looking lighter and brighter! If, however, you are finding your energy levels are lagging, it could be that you have cut your food intake too much, particularly your intake of carbohydrates. Focus on the following goals this week:

FOOD GOAL

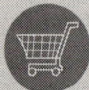

Ensure you are eating enough carbohydrate (from low-GI sources) to give you the energy to sustain your increased exercise and activity levels.

EXERCISE GOAL

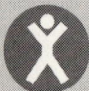

Aim to walk for a total of 30 minutes on six days at the same brisk pace as last week (around level 5 of the PRE scale) for the middle 15 minutes. *Plus* try to complete each of the resistance workouts, focusing on the upper and lower body respectively, three times during the week.

ACTIVITY GOAL

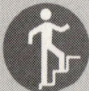

Instead of heading to the local automatic car wash, do it yourself by hand, including an internal spring clean.

FOOD FOR THOUGHT

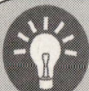

Facts and fallacies about the GI.

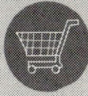

> ## FOOD GOAL
>
> Ensure you are eating enough carbohydrate (from low-GI sources) to give you the energy to sustain your increased activity and exercise levels.

While cutting out carbs might seem to bring rapid results when you weigh yourself, such weight loss is inevitably too difficult to maintain long term. You need a certain amount of carbs to function at your best, particularly given your recent increased exercise and activity levels.

Focus this week on the carb-rich foods you are eating and assess whether you are including a low-GI carb in each meal. Your goal is not to load your body with a huge amount of carbohydrate in one meal, but to spread a moderate amount of slowly absorbed low-GI carbs to fuel your body across the course of the day. This translates into gentle fluctuations in your blood glucose with less insulin being required to deal with the day's intake. Perhaps keep a diary for a few days and look back to check on how you are really doing. If you find you are not spreading your carb intake across the day, try following our suggested meal plans for a few days.

Sample day (low-GI choices are shown in bold)

Breakfast: **natural muesli** with **low-fat milk** and sliced **fresh berries**

Snack: **banana** and a **low-fat yoghurt**

Lunch: **lentil** soup with **low-GI bread** and reduced-fat cheese

Snack: hot chocolate made with **low-fat milk** and an **oatmeal biscuit**

Main meal: grilled salmon fillet with white bean mash and a green salad

EXERCISE GOAL

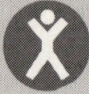

Aim to walk for a total of 30 minutes on six days at the same brisk pace as last week (around level 5 of the PRE scale) for the middle 15 minutes. *Plus* try to complete each of the resistance workouts, focusing on the upper and lower body respectively, three times during the week.

Most health authorities around the world agree that for health we should aim to achieve 30 minutes of walking on most days of the week. This week our goal is to meet those recommendations. You are now well on your way to better health, a leaner body and more active mind—well done!

Resistance exercises

Workout 1	Lower body exercises	'Core' strength abdominals and back
	Squats 1 set of 20	Full hover 2 × 30 seconds
	Lunges 10 each leg	Pointer 10 each side
	Power lunge 20 alternate legs	
Workout 2	**Upper body exercises**	
	Three-quarter push-ups 1 set of 20	Leg extensions 10 each leg
	Standing tricep extensions 1 set of 20	Ab curl 1 set of 20
	Bicep curl 1 set of 20	Oblique curl 20 each side

NEW EXERCISES

Three-quarter push-ups

This uses the same technique as the assisted push-ups (pages 71–72), but we make things a little more challenging by removing the help of the table (or stair). Ensure you set up with a wide hand stance and keep your bottom tucked while you lower your chest to the floor.

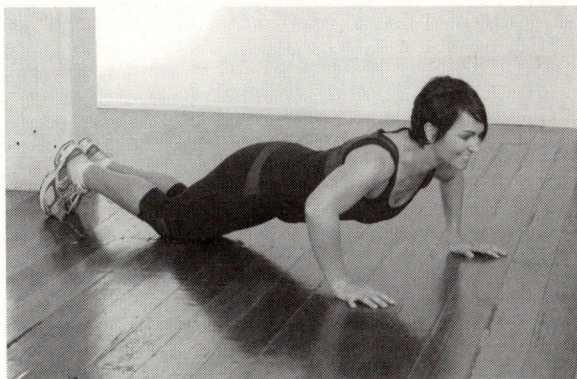

Oblique curl

This is a variation of the ab curl that you have already learnt (pages 114–115).

Strengthens and tones: waist and torso

How to do it:

1 From your ab curl position drop both knees down to the right.

2 Extend your left arm behind your body towards your left heel and reach for the heel as you curl the body up. Make sure you keep your shoulders square to the

ceiling (you will feel like twisting in the direction of your knees) and use your right hand to lightly support the weight of your head to avoid straining your neck.

3 Repeat on the other side.

How many: 20 curls on each side

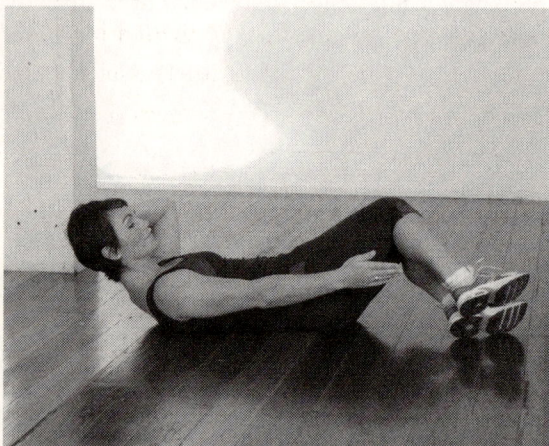

Sample diary

Monday	Tuesday	Wednesday	Thursday	Friday	Saturday	Sunday
30 min walk	30 min walk	30 min walk	30 min walk		30 min walk	30 min walk
+ workout 2	+ workout 1	+ workout 2	+ workout 1		+ workout 1	+ workout 2
40 mins	40 mins	40 mins	40 mins		40 mins	40 mins

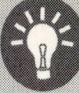

FOOD FOR THOUGHT
Facts and fallacies about the GI.

1 Carrots have a high GI

No, they don't! They have a GI of 39 and you can eat them as a 'free food'. The reason for the confusion: the first value ever published gave them a high GI (92). Unfortunately it was based on too few subjects and the resulting average was skewed. This error made the GI concept highly controversial right from the beginning.

2 The GI doesn't consider the amount of carbohydrate in a serving of food

That's true—it is a measure of the carbohydrate quality, not quantity. Do we need to know the quantity, too? For the most part, no. If you substitute a low-GI bread for others, a low-GI breakfast cereal for others and a low-GI rice for others, then you are achieving your goal: a low-GI diet in which the carbs are slowly digested and absorbed. If you are choosing chocolate over watermelon (not a good idea really) then it is sensible to consider both quality and quantity (the glycemic load).

3 Some foods have a high GI but contain little carbohydrate

True, there is a handful of foods that contain so little carbohydrate that their GI is irrelevant. This includes watermelon and rockmelon, pumpkin, parsnips and broadbeans. You can ignore their high GI.

4 Glycemic load (GL) makes more sense than GI

Not true. The GI can be more important than the GL. That's because it is critical to choose slowly digested carbs (low-GI carbs) over quickly digested ones (high-GI carbs), even if the GL is the same. You'll stay fuller for longer if you choose a normal portion of pasta (a low-GI food) over a small serve of potato (a high-GI food). Our primary goal should be improving the quality of the carbs (exchanging high GI for low GI), not reducing the quantity of carbohydrate eaten. A secondary goal—it's up to you—is to replace some of the high-GI carbs with good fats or lean protein.

5 Cutting carbs is the best way to lower insulin levels

No, that's not correct. While it is true that high-GI carbs produce high insulin responses, low-GI carbs have the same insulin demand as high-protein foods that contain no carbs. Moreover, people who eat more carbs have better insulin sensitivity than low-carb eaters.

6 Wholemeal products have low GI values

Not true most of the time. Wholemeal cereal products, especially those derived from wheat, usually have the same GI as their white counterparts. For example, white bread's GI is 70, wholemeal bread's GI is 71. One rule to follow is that if you can't see the grains it's probably not low GI, whatever it says on the packet. When wheat bran is finely milled, digestive enzymes can attack fast. That's not to say wholemeal cereals are unhealthy. There is good evidence that wholemeal foods improve insulin sensitivity and reduce disease risk. The best choices are both low GI and high in fibre.

7 The GI doesn't work in mixed meals

Yes, it does—it works perfectly. Why the controversy? Early studies on the subject of mixed meals were carried out by vocal opponents of the GI concept. Subsequent studies—at least a dozen from all over the world—proved convincingly that the GI of single foods could be used to predict the GI of a mixed meal. Moreover, long-term studies comparing high and low-GI diets show differences in measures of blood glucose control. If the GI values of single foods were not a good guide to food choices, then those differences would not be evident.

8 The GI doesn't work when you add protein or fat

Not true. When you add protein or fat to a high carbohydrate food—for example, add cheese to bread—the blood glucose response will go down. But if you then exchange the source of carbohydrate (instead of bread with cheese, you have pasta with cheese), then you can expect an even lower response. The relative ranking of carbohydrate foods according to their GI predicts the overall glycemic response even in the presence of extra protein and fat. There will be limits to this, of course—if your meal contains a lot of protein and fat and little in the way of carbs, then the GI becomes irrelevant.

9 Too many variables affect the blood glucose response to meals

It's true that there are many variables that affect your glycemic response to meals. But that criticism applies equally well to carbohydrate 'counting' as it does to the GI. And carbohydrate counting is highly recommended for people with diabetes. Your day-to-day variation will be influenced by many things, including things you did the day before: amount of exercise; consumption of fat, fibre and alcohol; and even amount of sleep. What's good to know is that a low-GI meal at dinner or breakfast will improve your glycemic response to lunch the following day, irrespective of what you eat.

10 Choosing low GI takes precedence over any other consideration

Of course not! If you're under the illusion that chocolate's low GI is a reason to go to town on it, then think again. In recommending the GI, we don't want people to throw commonsense to the wind. The GI is not meant to be used in isolation. Reducing saturated and trans fats is vitally important. Eat lots of fruit and vegies (bar potatoes) for their vitamins, minerals, anti-oxidants and fibre. Disregard their GI except in the case of potato. Cutting down on the volume of soft drinks, ice-cream, cakes, biscuits and confectionery, irrespective of their GI, is important. That does not mean strict avoidance—remember, an indulgence a day keeps bingeing at bay. That's especially true if your indulgence is low GI to boot.

'The great thing about the low-GI diet is that it is not restrictive. It has given me more freedom in what I eat and more energy.' – Veronica

I lost almost 20 kilos on the low-GI diet. I had tried various diets before, low fat, detox, etc. but it never made any difference to my weight and they were often quite restrictive in what they allowed you to eat. So I could never keep them up for long. It took one year to lose the weight, with once-a-week exercise, and now two years later I still have not regained the weight. My diet is varied, enjoyable and does not make me gain weight. The great thing about the low-GI diet is that it is not restrictive, you can eat most foods; you only need to modify your diet slightly, like eating grainy bread instead of white bread. I find low-GI foods taste better too. (Oat biscuits are great!) It has also allowed me to eat lots of foods that I would never have eaten before as I thought they were too fattening. It has given me more freedom in what I eat and more energy.

Week 9 Menu Plan

	BREAKFAST	SNACK	
MONDAY	Natural muesli topped with sliced banana and natural yoghurt	Low-fat drinking yoghurt	
TUESDAY	Grainy toast with a skim of peanut butter	Low-fat flavoured milk	
WEDNESDAY	A low-GI cereal with low-fat milk and sliced strawberries	A pear	
THURSDAY	Bircher muesli with sliced peach	A quarter of a honeydew melon	
FRIDAY	Natural muesli with 1 tablespoon of blueberries and natural yoghurt	A small handful of almonds	
SATURDAY	Banana and Ricotta Toasts (see page 265)	A handful of pistachio nuts in their shells	
SUNDAY	Scrambled eggs with grainy toast, grilled tomato and dry-fried mushrooms	A quarter of a rockmelon	

LUNCH	SNACK	DINNER
Sushi rolls and a bowl of miso soup	Apple slices and a chunk of reduced-fat cheddar	Lentil dhal with tandoori chicken, steamed Basmati rice and a tomato salad
Turkey and Peach Salsa Wraps (see page 230)	A quarter of a melon	Penne pasta stir-fried with smoked salmon, olives, spinach, halved cherry tomatoes, garlic and a little white wine
Pasta salad with corn, spring onion, capsicum, cherry tomatoes, olives and cucumber, and a little olive oil mayonnaise with sliced lean meat	Low-fat fruit yoghurt	Fajitas made with lean beef or chicken and capsicum. Serve with flour tortillas, salsa, guacamole, shredded lettuce, grated reduced-fat cheese and natural yoghurt
Pita bread with felafel, hummus and tabbouli	Carrot and celery sticks with tzatziki dip	Stir-fry with prawns, vegies and Hokkien noodles
Asian-style clear soup with noodles and seafood or chicken	A handful of cherries	Grilled or barbecued lamb kebabs served with tzatziki, spinach salad and grilled pita bread slices
Open sandwich on toasted pumpernickel bread with ham, low-fat cream cheese and salad vegies	A quarter of a melon	Grilled sardines with mixed bean salsa (can of mixed beans, spring onion, fresh coriander, lemon juice, olives, olive oil and halved cherry tomatoes) and a rocket salad
Roast lamb or beef with low-fat gravy and baked sweet potato, parsnip, beetroot, zucchini and carrot	An apple	Bowl of vegetable and bean soup with grainy bread

Week 10

The drive to consume a certain volume of food each day is heavily ingrained in human behaviour. We tend to consume the same physical bulk of food, regardless of its kilojoule content. Therefore, if the food we choose is energy dense—a little bit contains lots of kilojoules (think biscuits)—then it is very easy to overconsume. For this reason, it is critical to lower the energy density of our diet if we want to control our weight.

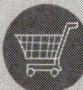

FOOD GOAL
Lowering the energy density of your diet.

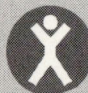

EXERCISE GOAL
Aim to walk for a total of 30 minutes on six days, at the same brisk pace as last week (around level 5 of the PRE scale) for the middle 15 minutes. *Plus* try to complete each of the resistance workouts, focusing on the upper and lower body respectively, three times during the week.

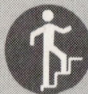

ACTIVITY GOAL
Try out a new active hobby. For example, join a dancing class—ballroom, salsa, line dancing, Scottish dancing or jazz; go rollerblading in the park; book in for golf lessons; or take your dog to agility classes.

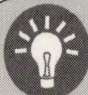

FOOD FOR THOUGHT
Incidental exercise—a lesson from the past.

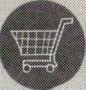

> ## FOOD GOAL
> Lowering the energy density of your diet.

Reducing the energy density of your diet will help you reduce your energy intake, and thereby facilitate weight loss. Energy density is a measure of how many kilojoules are contained in a food. Foods with a high energy density contain a large number of kilojoules in only a small amount of food. Chocolate is one example (22 kilojoules per gram). Foods of low energy density provide few calories for a large quantity of food. Apples have a low energy density (2 kilojoules per gram).

This week we encourage you to examine the energy density of foods that you regularly eat, with the aim of reducing the overall energy density of your diet. If you haven't looked at it before, start taking a look at the nutrition information panel on foods and work out their energy density. To calculate energy density, divide the energy (kilojoules) per 100 grams of the food by 100. A food can be considered energy dense if it has more than 5 kilojoules per gram.

Sample nutrition information panel

Nutrient	Per 100 g
Energy (kJ)	1500
Protein (g)	9.5
Fat—total (g)	3.0
—saturated (g)	1.1
Carbohydrate (g)	72.2
—sugars (g)	5.4

This food has an energy density of 1500 kilojoules per 100 grams = 15 kilojoules per gram. It has a high energy density.

Note that even though a food may be low in fat, it can still be high in energy density. High-fat foods will obviously be energy dense, but many commercial low-fat foods are high in energy density too, for example:

Energy density (kJ/100 g) of some popular low-fat foods	
Yoghurt, low-fat, fruit	3
Bananas	4
Bread, white	10
Wheat biscuit breakfast cereal	14
Cornflakes	16
Pretzels	16
Rice crackers	17
Plain, sweet biscuits	19

How to reduce the energy density of your diet

- Combine small servings of nutritious but energy-dense foods (such as nuts, cheese and olive oil) with larger servings of low energy-dense foods (such as fruit, vegetables, pasta, rice and grainy breads).
- Base meals on vegetables and legumes using meat as an accompaniment and nuts as a condiment.
- Use oils (such as olive oil) where they will increase your enjoyment of low energy-dense foods (especially plant foods and fish) by improving the flavour of such dishes (for example, salads with dressing, roasted vegetables and

panfried fish). Added oils may also help your absorption of fat-soluble nutrients and phytochemicals from plant foods.

- Minimise foods containing hidden animal fats (fatty meat, full-fat dairy products, some fast/processed food) and hydrogenated plant fats (some fast/processed food, commercial cakes/biscuits).
- Avoid eating large volumes of low-fat but energy-dense foods, particularly commercially processed cereals and biscuits.
- Eat more fruit and vegetables. Large amounts of low energy-dense foods such as fruit and vegetables help to 'dilute' the energy density of your diet.
  —Add extra vegetables (frozen if you prefer) to stir-fried meat, chicken, prawns, fish or tofu.
  —Eat salad daily.
  —Include salad ingredients in sandwiches and rolls.
  —Throw some vegies onto the barbecue with meat. Try zucchini, corn cobs, capsicum, mushrooms, eggplant or thick slices of parboiled sweet potato or onion. (Use vegetable oil spray on a cold grill or a little olive oil to prevent sticking.)
  —Try a vegetarian main dish at least once a week.
  —For quick munching, keep celery, capsicum, baby carrots, cucumber, broccoli or cauliflower florets and cherry or grape tomatoes on hand.

Take care not to *over*estimate how much you do or *under*estimate how much you eat.

EXERCISE GOAL

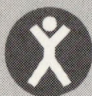

Aim to walk for a total of 30 minutes on six days, at the same brisk pace as last week (around level 5 of the PRE scale) for the middle 15 minutes. *Plus* try to complete each of the resistance workouts, focusing on the upper and lower body respectively, three times during the week.

Resistance exercises

Workout 1	Lower body exercises	'Core' strength abdominals and back
	Squats 1 set of 20	Full hover 2×30 seconds
	Squats with alternate leg extension 10 each leg	Pointer 10 each side
	Power lunge 20 alternating legs	
Workout 2	Upper body exercises	
	Three-quarter push-ups 1 set of 20	Leg extensions 10 each leg
	Standing tricep extensions 1 set of 20	Ab curl 1 set of 20
	Bicep curl 1 set of 20	Oblique curl 20 each side

NEW EXERCISE

Squats with alternate leg extension

This advanced exercise really targets the bottom by adding a lift at the top of the squat. If possible, use a mirror to help you perfect your technique and avoid leaning to one side as you lift.

Strengthens and tones: legs and bottom

How to do it:

1 Perform your squat as before (see pages 59–60), but as you rise, extend one leg at a 45-degree angle behind you, squeezing your bottom muscles as you do so.

2 Ensure that you maintain good posture by pulling in your navel and lifting your chest. Avoid swinging your leg—rather try for a controlled fluid movement without arching the back.

3 Repeat, lifting alternate legs each time.

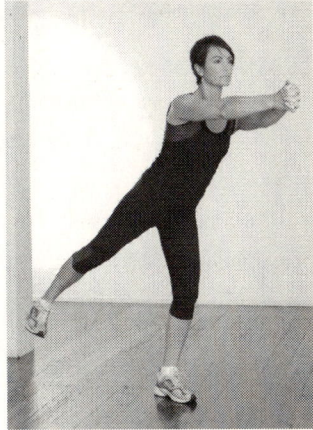

How many: 20, using alternate legs each time

Sample diary

Monday	Tuesday	Wednesday	Thursday	Friday	Saturday	Sunday
30 min walk	30 min walk	30 min walk	30 min walk		30 min walk	30 min walk
+ workout 1	+ workout 2	+ workout 1	+ workout 2		+ workout 1	+ workout 2
40 mins	40 mins	40 mins	40 mins		40 mins	40 mins

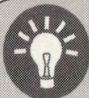

FOOD FOR THOUGHT

Incidental exercise—a lesson from the past.

Life today is far more challenging on our brains than it is on our bodies. Technology has made many of the everyday arduous tasks our grandparents would have done by hand far easier and less time consuming. Washing machines, dishwashers, automatic car washes, drive-through food outlets, shopping malls and the internet all make life easier. The result, however, has been that modern life makes it very difficult for us to control our weight. Imagine living one day without any of this technology—washing your clothes or scrubbing the floor by hand, walking to the shops, walking home carrying heavy bags, chopping logs for the fire, creating everything you eat from the raw ingredients and washing up by hand.

Perhaps you still do some of these things, but imagine every day being filled with this level of activity. In addition to the high levels of activity in the past, food was not so readily available or so appetising—the wide choice of foods we have now encourages us to eat more. You can see that our environment works against our ability to control our weight. While no one wants to see a return to washing by hand and chopping wood for the fire, we can take a lesson from the past and aim to become more active each and every day.

Consider your own lifestyle and environment and think about where you could build in a little more activity. It doesn't have to be much and it probably won't feel like much at the time, but all those little movements add up to a considerable increase in your energy output over the coming weeks, months and years.

Some suggestions to build activity naturally into your days

At home

- Wash the car by hand.
- Iron while you watch television.
- Spend 20 minutes gardening.
- Mow the lawn.
- Clean one set of windows.
- Walk the dog.
- Stroll to your local shops.
- Spend an afternoon window shopping.
- Play with the kids.
- Vacuum the floor.

At work

- Use the printer along the hall or, even better, one floor up or down.
- Get up from your desk to speak with a colleague rather than use email.
- Stand and stretch while on the telephone.
- Go outside at lunchtime for a stroll—walking while shopping still counts!
- Use the upstairs or downstairs lavatory.
- Volunteer to buy the cappuccinos.
- Find an excuse to deliver something somewhere.
- Meeting with a colleague? Why not walk while you talk.

Week 10 Menu Plan

	BREAKFAST	SNACK	
MONDAY	Half a grapefruit followed by low-GI toast with avocado and sliced tomato	A handful of peanuts in their shell	
TUESDAY	Natural muesli with sliced apple and low-fat milk	Oatmeal biscuits with hummus	
WEDNESDAY	Carton of low-fat flavoured milk and a banana	Slice of raisin toast with low-fat cream cheese	
THURSDAY	Mixed nut bar, an apple and a low-fat yoghurt	Oatmeal biscuit and a skim milk cappuccino	
FRIDAY	Toasted grainy bread with ricotta cheese and fruit jam	A handful of red grapes	
SATURDAY	Poached egg with smoked salmon, toasted sourdough and spinach	A small glass of orange juice	
SUNDAY	Low-fat yoghurt with fruit salad and a sprinkle of mixed nuts and seeds	A glass of vegetable juice	

LUNCH	SNACK	DINNER
Tuna Rice Paper Rolls (see page 231)	A nectarine	Chickpea and vegetable curry with steamed Basmati rice
Bowl of vegetable soup with grainy crackers and low-fat cream cheese	A peach	Stir-fried greens with a grilled chicken breast and spiced lentils
Salad with a can of tuna, a handful of mixed beans and a little yoghurt dressing	Six raw Brazil nuts	Tortillas with refried beans, lettuce, salsa, chicken strips and natural yoghurt
Grainy bread with toasted reduced-fat cheese and tomato	An apple	Spinach and ricotta lasagne with a large green salad
Indian Chicken Burgers (see page 233) with hot chilli salsa, warmed pita bread and shredded lettuce	Natural yoghurt with blueberries	Grilled lean steak with mashed sweet potato, steamed greens and carrots
Grainy crackers with cottage cheese, cucumber and sliced tomato and a cup of ready-to-serve soup	A handful of dried apricots	Asian-style noodle and seafood stir-fry with plenty of mixed vegies
Grainy bread sandwich with hard-boiled egg, olive oil mayonnaise and salad	Fruit Parfaits (see page 266)	Roast chicken with baked vegies—sweet potato, beetroot, carrot, pumpkin and squash. Drizzle with olive oil and balsamic vinegar and bake for 30 minutes

Week 11

This week, focus on these goals:

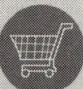

FOOD GOAL

Making the best of takeaway.

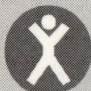

EXERCISE GOAL

This week we split the walks into one shorter, brisker walk (30 minutes maintaining a brisk pace of level 5 for 20 minutes) and one longer but gentler walk (40 minutes at a steady pace of level 4). Aim to complete each walk three times. *Plus* try to complete the full resistance workout, incorporating both upper and lower body exercises, three times during the week.

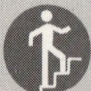

ACTIVITY GOAL

Whenever you are on a bus or a train for a short journey, choose to stand rather than sit.

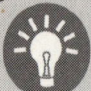

FOOD FOR THOUGHT

Can takeaway food be part of a healthy diet?

FOOD GOAL

Making the best of takeaway.

Who said takeaway food can't be good for you? It definitely isn't if you eat it every night, but you can certainly put together a reasonable meal in minimal time with some astute choices and a little help from your local takeaway provider. You will need to think about frequency, however, and that is one of the goals this week. How often is it reasonable for you or your family to be eating takeaway foods for the main meal? Some would say once a month, others would say twice a week; we suggest no more than once or twice a week.

The other thing to think about is what you order. We'd like you to practise putting together a balanced meal with takeaway food this week. Here are some examples using our three-step guide to planning a balanced meal.

Planning a balanced meal with takeway food

Low-GI carb	Fruit and vegetables	Protein and good fats
Home-cooked Doongara CleverRice or Moolgiri medium grain	Stir-fry vegetables	Braised beef and cashew nuts
Basmati rice and lentil dhal	Home-prepared green salad	Tandoori chicken
Corn cobs	Home-prepared coleslaw with canola dressing	Barbecued chicken minus the skin

EXERCISE GOAL

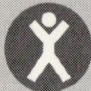

This week we split the walks into one shorter, brisker walk (30 minutes maintaining a brisk pace of level 5 for 20 minutes) and one longer but gentler walk (40 minutes at a steady pace of level 4). Aim to complete each walk three times. *Plus* try to complete the full resistance workout, incorporating both upper and lower body exercises, three times during the week.

Resistance exercises

This week we are going to combine the resistance training exercises into one effective workout to be undertaken three times in the week. We suggest you do the workout on the days you complete your 30-minute walk to give you more time on the other three days for a longer walk. Maximising your time in this way means that you never need to spend hours exercising yet continue to work towards your goals.

Lower body exercises	
Squats	1 set of 20
Squats with alternate leg extension	1 set of 20
Lunges	10 each leg
Power lunges	20 alternating legs

Upper body exercises	
Three-quarter push-ups	1 set of 20
Standing tricep extensions	1 set of 20
Bicep curl	1 set of 20

'Core' strength, abdominals and back	
Full hover	1 x 30 seconds
Pointer	10 each side
Leg extensions	10 each leg
Ab curl	1 set of 20
Oblique curl	20 each side

Sample diary

Monday	Tuesday	Wednesday	Thursday	Friday	Saturday	Sunday
40 min walk 2	30 min walk 1	40 min walk 2	30 min walk 1		40 min walk 2	30 min walk 1
	+ resistance workout		+ resistance workout			+ resistance workout
40 mins	50 mins	40 mins	50 mins		40 mins	50 mins

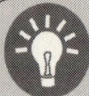

FOOD FOR THOUGHT

Can takeaway food be part of a healthy diet?

Most people eat takeaway *sometimes*. That's okay; as we have said before, it is the frequency that matters. The real problem exists for *some* people who eat takeaway *most* of the time. With an average meal from a fast food restaurant supplying about half most people's daily energy requirements, those 'two for one' or 'upsize' meal deals, 'free fries' and 'delivered to your door' options really are better off resisted *most* of the time. So, decide on a reasonable, realistic limit for you and your family and stick to it.

On the plus side
- It is a welcome break from cooking.
- You can make upsize meals feed two people or one adult and a child.
- Kilojoule-conscious items now appear on some menus.
- You can add something nutritious (such as a salad or vegetables) at home.

On the minus side
- The menu is often limited.
- Foods are high in kilojoules, salt and saturated fat.
- Meal deals that upsize for a small cost trap you into increasing your kilojoule intake.
- The difference between a small and a large can be double the kilojoules.

- It takes so little time to eat the food from fast food restaurants (no or little chewing required)—all those kilojoules, and you are not even feeling full.
- Even just a muffin and coffee can set you back 2000 kilojoules (that is a third of the day's requirement for some people).

For our suggestions on what to choose when ordering, see pages 195–200.

Here are some more healthy takeaway options and quick-prep home alternatives:

- A regular hamburger with salad—hold the high-kilojoule extras such as cheese and bacon
- Salad sandwiches and rolls with ham, salmon, silverside or egg included
- Vegetarian pizza (thin crust)—teamed with a tossed salad
- Takeaway pasta with anything other than a creamy sauce
- Oven-heat fish and chips or wedges from the freezer—check for the varieties cooked in healthy oil—served with vegetables and salad
- Vegetarian lasagne
- Fresh noodles added to pre-cut stir-fry vegetable mix (fresh or frozen) with prawns
- Canned mexican beans on low-salt corn chips with dollops of avocado
- Chunks of skinless barbecued chicken added to a packet of chicken noodle soup with egg vermicelli, canned cream corn, frozen baby peas and shallots to make a chicken and corn soup
- Vegetarian kebabs.

Week 11 Menu Plan

	BREAKFAST	SNACK	
MONDAY	Grilled lean bacon served on a slice of toasted sourdough and topped with sliced tomato	A banana	
TUESDAY	Toasted cheese and tomato sandwich from the takeaway shop and an apple	A cup of cherries	
WEDNESDAY	Toasted grainy bread topped with a little peanut butter and sliced banana	An apple	
THURSDAY	Fruit salad with natural yoghurt and a small handful of mixed nuts and seeds	A skim milk cappuccino and oatmeal biscuit	
FRIDAY	On the run: a nut and seed bar and an apple	Low-fat fruit yoghurt	
SATURDAY	Scrambled egg with smoked salmon and spinach on a slice of toasted grainy bread	A pear	
SUNDAY	Breakfast barley: cover the barley with water and simmer for 30–40 minutes until soft. Towards the end of cooking add a mixture of dried fruit, nuts and seeds and serve with warmed low-fat milk	An apple	

LUNCH	SNACK	DINNER
Felafel roll with felafel, tabbouli and hummus	A nectarine	Lamb salad with tzatziki: grill or barbecue a lean lamb fillet and slice. Serve on a large salad of baby spinach leaves, semi-dried tomatoes, olives, cucumber and capsicum. Drizzle with tzatziki
Mixed sushi box and miso soup	A small handful of raw almonds	Thai green chicken curry with a bag of Asian stir-fried frozen vegies added at home and served with home-cooked Doongara CleverRice
Multigrain bread sandwich of cream cheese, smoked salmon and snowpea sprouts with salad	A low-fat fruit yoghurt	Barbecued chicken, skin removed and meat chopped, added to a pot of chicken stock with long noodles, creamed corn and shallots
Combination long soup	Low-fat flavoured milk	Mexican-style bean burrito with steamed Basmati or Doongara CleverRice, salsa and a green salad
Roast beef open sandwich on rye sourdough with plenty of salad vegies	A peach	Grilled fish fillet with a handful of chips, vinegar and a rocket salad
Lentil, Beetroot and Feta Salad (see page 234)	A handful of pistachios in their shells	Beef and vegetable stir-fry in black bean sauce with Hokkien noodles
Sunday Roast with mashed sweet potato and steamed green peas, carrots and brussels sprouts	Creamed Rice with Rhubarb and Strawberries (see page 268)	Vegetable soup with melted cheese on toast

Week 12

You have made major changes over the last three months and you should be feeling the rewards of your hard efforts. Now is the time to start reinforcing all the changes you have made and making sure that none of your old habits are sneaking back in on a regular basis. Focus on the following goals this week:

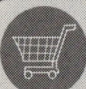

FOOD GOAL

Making healthy eating a habit.

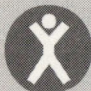

EXERCISE GOAL

As last week, aim to complete a shorter, brisker walk (30 minutes, maintaining a brisk pace of level 5 for 20 minutes) on three days, and one longer but gentler walk (40 minutes at a steady pace of level 4) on three days. *Plus* try to complete the full resistance workout, incorporating more advanced exercises for the upper and lower body, three times during the week.

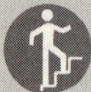

ACTIVITY GOAL

Become an active person by nature where you see every moment as an opportunity for movement. In other words, be the person who offers to run an errand, walk to the local shop for the papers, walk the dog or carry the shopping home. Every moment of activity counts in the long run.

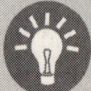

FOOD FOR THOUGHT

Helping yourself towards healthier eating habits.

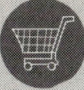

There is no magic bullet for permanent weight loss, but people who have lost weight and maintained it over the long haul reveal that weight-loss maintainers:

- Have a positive attitude towards changing their diet to improve health
- Possess a willingness to lose weight slowly
- Make lasting changes to their diet and exercise patterns
- Feel comfortable with, rather than restricted by, dietary changes.

So how are you feeling about what you have done so far? It is time to reassess your eating habits with another food diary, to see how far you have come. As in Week 1, write down everything you eat and drink each day and compare it with the diary you first kept. Hopefully you will see some major differences. The aim is to keep it going! Remember, success is not about achieving a particular weight, but changing the way you eat and live. It is the simple changes made every day to the way we shop, cook, prepare and eat that can change our lives.

Motivation is what gets you started. Habit is what keeps you going.

EXERCISE GOAL

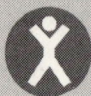

As last week, aim to complete a shorter, brisker walk (30 minutes, maintaining a brisk pace of level 5 for 20 minutes) on three days, and one longer but gentler walk (40 minutes at a steady pace of level 4) on three days. *Plus* try to complete the full resistance workout, incorporating more advanced exercises for the upper and lower body, three times during the week.

Resistance exercises

You should be feeling more energetic, alive and starting to reap the rewards of all your efforts over the last weeks. This week we make the resistance exercises a little more challenging to ensure your body keeps changing.

Lower body exercises	
Squats	1 set of 20
Squats with alternate leg extension	1 set of 20
Lunges	10 each leg
Power lunges	20 alternating legs
Upper body exercises	
Full push-ups	1 set of 10
Tricep push-ups	2 sets of 10
Bicep curl	1 set of 20
'Core' strength, abdominals and back	
Full hover	2 x 30 seconds
Pointer	10 each side
Leg extensions	10 each leg
Ab curl	1 set of 20
Oblique curl	20 each side

NEW EXERCISES

Full push-ups

Challenge yourself by increasing the load your body has to lift by performing your push-ups on your toes. As before, be sure to keep your bottom in line with your body (see page 147).

How many: Try to complete 10 full push-ups, then, if you need to, lower your knees to complete the second set of 10 in the kneeling position.

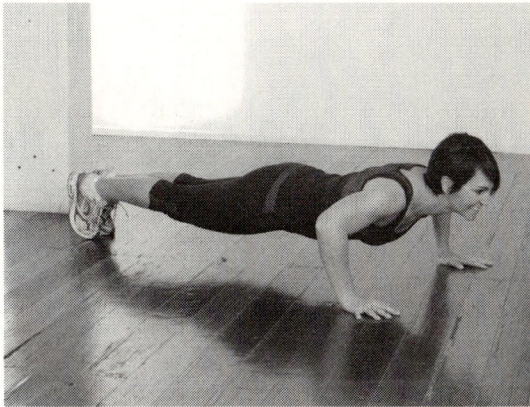

Tricep push-ups

This is a more challenging exercise for the triceps than the standing extensions because your resistance in the push-up is coming from your own body weight, which is undoubtedly heavier than the weight you have been using.

Strengthens and tones: back of the arm and shoulders

How to do it:

1 From your regular three-quarter push-up position (see page 147), step your hands in closer until they are directly under your shoulders. You may find it more comfortable to make a fist rather than a flat hand as this allows you to keep your wrist straighter.

2 Lower your chest towards the floor and back, with your elbows tracking close to your ribcage.

How many: Try to complete 2 sets of 10 with a short rest in between.

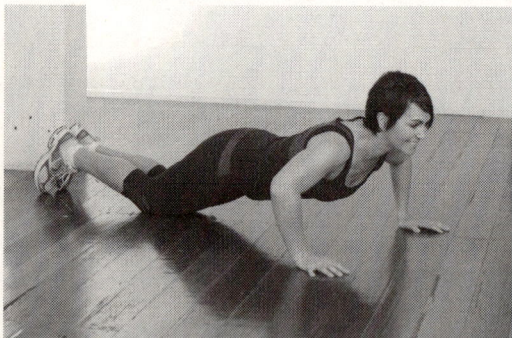

Sample diary

Monday	Tuesday	Wednesday	Thursday	Friday	Saturday	Sunday
40 min walk 2	30 min walk 1	40 min walk 2	30 min walk 1		40 min walk 2	30 min walk 1
	+ resistance workout		+ resistance workout			+ resistance workout
40 mins	50 mins	40 mins	50 mins		40 mins	40 mins

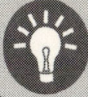

FOOD FOR THOUGHT
Helping yourself towards healthier eating habits.

1 Listen to your appetite

The most normal way to eat is in response to your appetite. The first step for some people is tuning in to it, eating when they are hungry and stopping when they feel full (not stuffed). It may help you to know that it is normal to eat more on some days and less on others.

2 Become aware of non-hungry eating

Eating is an extremely complex behaviour. There is a lot more to it than simply satisfying hunger or meeting nutrient needs. Food is part of socialising and celebrating, comforting and boredom filling. We eat food that is offered so as not to offend a host, we eat because we feel anxious or depressed, we finish off what the kids have left rather than waste it, we eat just because it looks good, or because it is there. All this non-hungry eating isn't wrong but it can contribute to overeating and we need to be aware of it if we are to do anything about it.

3 Eat regularly

Have you ever noticed that the hungrier you are the more tempting high-kilojoule foods such as chocolate, biscuits and chips are? And the harder it is to stop at one? You will find it easier to eat normally and control your appetite by regularly grazing on low-GI smart carbs.

4   Think about what to eat, rather than what not to eat
What happens if I ask you not to think of a pink
elephant? You imagine it, right? The future is what we
imagine, so rather than thinking of what you don't
want to eat, think of what you do.

5   Make overeating as difficult as possible
When you go to have a slice of bread, take out one
slice, then seal up the bag and put the loaf away. Put
the spreads and toppings away before you sit down to
eat. Out of sight generally means out of mind. Keep
those occasional foods out of sight but, better still,
don't buy them routinely.

6   Make healthy foods more accessible
Put healthy foods where you will find them first:
* Washed, shiny apples and stone fruits in an attractive
  bowl in the fridge
* Dried fruit and nuts in an airtight jar on your bench
  or desk
* Pre-sliced tomato and cucumber in the fridge, ready
  to use on sandwiches or crackers
* Tubs of low-fat yoghurt in the fridge
* A loaf of fruit bread by the toaster

These are just a few of the ways you can increase your
chances of eating the types of foods you planned to
eat.

7   Don't prepare enough to have leftovers
If you cook too much and have leftovers, serve them
into containers and put them in the fridge before you

sit down to eat the main meal. Still finding yourself tempted to go back for seconds? Try brushing your teeth soon after finishing a meal.

8 **Minimise other distractions while you are eating**
Sitting in front of the television with a bag of chips or a block of chocolate, it is very easy to absentmindedly finish the lot. Focus on and savour what you are eating.

9 **Stick to regular times for your meals and snacks**
When you find yourself thinking about eating outside of your usual meal and snack times, try these four steps:
- Delay.
- Deep breathe.
- Drink water.
- Do something else.

10 **Put some thought and planning into your meals**
Preparing food is, for most of us, a necessity to eating, a fact of life. So take the time to cook—go to a class if you don't know how. Try different foods, write a shopping list, buy foods in season, get to know your local shopkeepers, shop regularly and develop a passion for good, healthy food.

Think about what to eat, rather than what not to eat.

Week 12 Menu Plan

	BREAKFAST	SNACK	
MONDAY	High-fibre cereal with sliced banana and low-fat milk	Fruit snack pack	
TUESDAY	Toasted sourdough with avocado, smoked mackerel and sliced tomato	Fruit salad	
WEDNESDAY	Porridge with sliced banana, sultanas and low-fat milk	A slice of raisin toast with low-fat cream cheese	
THURSDAY	High-protein cereal with sliced strawberries and low-fat milk	Oatmeal biscuits	
FRIDAY	Boiled eggs with grainy toast soldiers	An orange	
SATURDAY	Half a grapefruit followed by grainy toast with reduced-fat cheese and sliced tomato	An apple	
SUNDAY	Spinach and mushroom omelette with a slice of toasted soy and linseed bread	A glass of carrot and orange juice	

LUNCH	SNACK	DINNER
Tuna sandwich on grainy bread with corn, olive oil mayonnaise and sliced cucumber	Low-fat fruit yoghurt	Mushroom and Vegetable Stir-fry (see page 254)
Lentil soup and a grainy roll	A handful of peanuts in their shell	Grilled lamb cutlets with sweet potato and pumpkin mash and steamed green beans, carrots and broccoli
Toasted grainy bread topped with a small can of baked beans and sliced tomato	A handful of grapes	Chicken breast baked in orange juice served with boiled new potatoes and stir-fried greens
Tomato soup with grainy bread and low-fat cheese	A quarter of a melon	Beef Kebabs with Vegetable Noodle Salad (see page 247)
Chicken and salad tortilla wrap	A low-fat drinking yoghurt	Vegetable and chickpea curry with Basmati rice
Ham, Corn and Zucchini Muffins (see page 227) with salad	Carrot sticks with hummus dip	Cover a whole fish with chopped garlic, ginger, coriander leaves and lemon juice and wrap in foil. Bake or barbecue for 30 minutes and serve with a large mixed salad
Grilled sardines (canned or fresh) on sourdough toast and tomato and avocado salsa	An apple	Pork and vegetable stir-fry in oyster sauce with Hokkien noodles

Daily food, television and activity diary

Make three enlarged photocopies and complete a three-day diary once a month to start with, then every three months in the first 12 months to help you focus on your strengths and weaknesses.

Date _____

Meal	Time	Food and drinks consumed (indicate item and amount)	Did you include (tick):			Situation How did you feel? (e.g. happy, sad, angry)
			Low-GI carbs?	Protein?	Good fats?	

TV duration *(circle)***:**
0   30   60   90   120   150   180   or more ____ minutes

Exercise type *(tick)***:** ☐ Aerobic   ☐ Resistance

Exercise duration *(circle)***:**
0   5   10   15   20   30   45   60   or more ____ minutes

Rate of perceived exertion *(circle)***:**
1   2   3   4   5   6   7   8   9   10

Chapter 4
Doing it for Life: Preventing Weight Regain

IN 'DOING IT FOR LIFE', OUR FOCUS TURNS FROM WEIGHT loss to weight maintenance, from 'holding your hand' to 'giving you the skills and knowledge' that will maximise your chances of successful long-term weight control. It is important you spend at least the next three months preventing weight regain (maintaining your current weight) before tackling further weight loss by repeating the 12-week program. This alternating three-month pattern of weight loss and weight maintenance takes the pressure off and gives your body time to adjust. The bottom line is that you need to remain focused on eating well and exercising regularly.

It is going to take *at least 12 months* of persistent effort to convert your old eating and lifestyle pattern into a new and healthy one. Unfortunately, many people mistakenly believe that once the desired amount of weight is lost, the hard part is over. Before they know it, they have regained the weight they lost, often in less time than it took to lose it and with added 'interest'.

Characteristics of long-term 'weight losers'

They have high levels of physical activity.

Their exercise is usually brisk walking but often includes weight lifting.

They use a pedometer to count steps per day (see page 208–09).

They watch the total amount of food eaten.

They eat a reduced fat, not low carb, diet.

They frequently 'self-monitor' (use diet and activity diaries).

Characteristics of weight regainers

They resume their old ways.

They relax their dietary restraint.

They reduce their physical activity.

Planning the right meals for weight maintenance

Your healthy low-GI diet will be easy to maintain because, unlike low carb or kilojoule-restricted diets, it is not an enormous departure from either the social or individual norm. Concentrating on the *quality* rather than *quantity* of carbs and fats gives you built-in flexibility and freedom.

Because you aren't trying to *lose* more weight, you can eat a little more each day. This could be an extra serve of fruit or low-fat dairy food, or both if you weigh more than 100 kilograms. You might even like to have an extra indulgence occasionally. But to achieve your goal and maintain your current weight, continue to base your food choices on the seven dietary guidelines of the low-GI diet. Here's a hot tip—adding an extra serve of protein in the form of lean meat, fish or chicken is especially helpful in preventing weight regain. On pages 188–91 we give you some ideas for building breakfasts, light meals and main meals around low-GI carbs. For more low-GI recipes and meal ideas check out *The Low GI Diet Cookbook* and *Low GI Diet Handbook*, both published by Hachette Australia.

To maintain your current weight:

- Base your food choices on the seven dietary guidelines of a low-GI diet.
- Eat seven or more servings of fruit and vegetables every day.
- Eat low-GI breads and cereals.
- Eat legumes, including soybeans, chickpeas and lentils, more often.
- Eat nuts more regularly.
- Eat more fish and seafood.
- Eat lean red meats, poultry and eggs.
- Eat low-fat dairy products.
- Listen to your body's cues for food intake and fine-tune your eating behaviour.
- Ensure that you are eating foods in the correct proportions using our three-step guide to meal planning:
  Start with a low-GI carbohydrate.
  Add a generous serve of vegetables or fruit.
  Plus add some protein with a little healthy fat for good measure.
- Make breakfast a priority. It recharges your brain and speeds up your metabolism after an overnight 'fast'.
- Maintain your exercise and activity program—this is the same activity level you achieved in Week 12.

Breakfasts

Low-GI + carb	Fruit and + vegetables	Protein and = good fat	Balanced low-GI meal
Muesli	Strawberries and yoghurt	Low-fat milk and yoghurt	Muesli with fruit
Baked beans	Mushrooms	Poached egg	Poached eggs, mushrooms and baked beans
Rolled oats	Raisins with banana slices	Low-fat milk	Raisin and banana porridge
Grainy toast	Fresh, ripe, sliced tomato and lettuce	Rindless eye bacon and a smear of barbecue sauce	BLT
Low-fat plain yoghurt with a drizzle of honey	Mashed ripe banana	Low-fat milk with a dash of nutmeg	Banana smoothie
Sourdough toast	Tomato juice	Herrings with a squeeze of lemon	Herrings on sourdough
Grainy toast	Sliced red apple	Reduced-fat cheddar	Toasted cheese and apple sandwiches
Low-fat vanilla yoghurt	Fresh chopped seasonal fruit	Mixed nuts and seeds	Fruit and nut yoghurt
Fruit toast	Fruit spread or fresh sliced stone fruit	Fresh ricotta cheese	Raisin toast with ricotta and fruit
Grainy toast	Shallots, mushrooms tomatoes and parsley	Eggs and grated reduced-fat cheese	Savoury omelette on toast

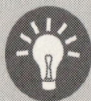

WATCH YOUR SERVING SIZES.

Listen to your appetite and let it guide how much you eat.

Light Meals

Low-GI carb	+ Fruit and vegetables	+ Protein and good fat	= Balanced low-GI meal
Sourdough bread	Lettuce, tomato, beetroot, onion	Minute steak	Steak sandwich
Flat bread	Tabbouli salad hummus	Felafel and kebab	Felafel roll
Sweetcorn cobs	Coleslaw	Barbecued chicken	Chicken and salad
Grainy bread	Lettuce, tomato, cucumber, beetroot, alfalfa, grated carrot and onion	Shaved ham	Ham and salad sandwich
Pasta	Napoletana sauce	Shaved parmesan cheese	Pasta Napoletana
Grainy bread	Sliced ripe tomatoes drizzled with olive oil and balsamic vinegar plus torn basil	Canned tuna (drained) combined with garlic, capers, parsley and olive oil, plus a little hummus to spread on the bread	Tuna tapenade and tomato salad
Mixed grain bread	Lettuce, cucumber and white onion	Red salmon, plus a little light cream cheese to spread on the bread	Salmon and lettuce sandwich
Toasted sourdough rubbed with a clove of garlic	Slow-roasted tomatoes and field mushrooms	Baked ricotta with herbed olive oil for dressing	Garlic toast with tomatoes, mushrooms and baked ricotta
Five bean mix with diced capsicum and shallots, tossed in oil, lemon and parsley	Salad greens, tomato, grated carrot and diced cucumber	Grated cheddar cheese	Cheese and bean salad

Main Meals

Low-GI + carb	Fruit and + vegetables	Protein and = good fat	Balanced low-GI meal
Corn tortilla with refried beans or Mexican beans	Shredded lettuce, tomato, diced celery and cucumber with tomato salsa	Lean minced beef, grated cheese and a dollop of mayonnaise for the salad	Beef and bean tortillas with salad
Canned brown lentils	Diced tomato, shredded English spinach and lemon juice	Lamb fillet marinated in olive oil, garlic and oregano	Barbecued Lamb with Lentil Salad and Yoghurt Dressing (see page 246)
Sweet potato	A bunch of rocket or mixed salad greens	Fillets of bream, ocean perch, flake or ling brushed with olive oil and black pepper	Sweet Potato Fish cakes (see page 232)
Basmati rice and dhal	Curry powder or paste plus cauliflower, carrot, green peas and canned tomatoes	Diced beef or lamb browned in canola oil with garlic and onion	Indian curry and rice
Baby new potatoes, steamed and cooled	Fresh green beans (blanched), cherry tomatoes (halved) and kalamata olives, dressed with olive oil and red wine vinegar	Canned tuna in water (drained) and hard-boiled egg (quartered)	Tuna salad
Sweet potato	Strips of red capsicum and red onion plus steamed green beans	Eggs	Vegetable Frittata (see page 225) with green beans

Low-GI carb +	Fruit and vegetables +	Protein and = good fat	Balanced low-GI meal
Canned borlotti beans	Canned tomatoes, onions, garlic, carrots, celery and swede	Lean diced beef browned in olive oil	Beef and bean casserole
Steamed Doongara CleverRice or Basmati rice or Moolgiri grain rice	Asian stir-fry frozen vegetable mix or fresh snowpeas, baby corn, carrot, onion and Asian greens	Chicken, beef, lamb or pork strips stir-fried in peanut oil with chilli plum sauce	Stir-fry with rice
Steamed corn on the cob	Mixed salad	Skinless barbecued chicken	Chicken with salad
Spaghetti	Onion, garlic, mushrooms and capsicum with a jar of tomato pasta sauce	Lean minced beef	Spaghetti bolognaise

Remember these: Ten tips for preventing weight regain

1 Never skip meals (or you will reduce your metabolic rate).
2 Eat a really good breakfast.
3 Eat at least three to four times a day.
4 Limit television to less than 12 hours per week.
5 Choose low-GI carbs at every meal.
6 Eat lean protein sources at every meal.
7 Don't skimp on the fats—just choose healthy ones.
8 Eat seven serves of fruit and vegies every day.
9 Schedule moderate physical activity for 30–60 minutes on six days out of seven.
10 One day a week, just relax and enjoy.

One meal for the whole family

Family support is a vital part of eating and living well. If one person in a household changes their eating habits, the whole household may have to adapt. Here are some tips for harmonious family eating and activity.

- Aim to prepare the same meal for the whole family.
- Eat dinner together.
- Involve others in food choices and meal planning.
- Make family lifestyle changes—take a stroll together after dinner, have a television-free night once a week, or try having meals outdoors.
- Don't buy food you want to avoid. If your kids are clamouring for foods that you are trying to avoid, give them the money that you would normally spend on those treats. Let them decide what they want to buy with it.
- Enjoy treats together when the occasion arises. Food is a traditional part of most celebrations and treats will be even more special if you reserve them for these times.

Growing good food habits in your children

1   Don't restrict their kilojoules.
2   Serve sensible portions (about the size of their fist).
3   Allow all foods, including desserts.
4   Involve them in shopping and food preparation.
5   Make a general rule: three bites of every food on the plate.
6   Limit soft drinks and fruit juices; replace with low-fat milk.
7   Don't keep soft drinks in the house; purchase them only outside the home.
8   Limit fast food to twice per week.

Eat well on weekends and holidays

One of the hardest places to make healthy choices is on the road. It might seem easy to pull into the 'drive-thru' for a bite to eat, but you will save money if you plan a proper stop. Choose from the menu sensibly and enjoy the break from routine.

Alternatively, if you know there is a rest stop or beauty spot en route, plan ahead and enjoy a roadside picnic. A lookout, walking track or park can give you the opportunity not only to refuel your batteries, but to stretch those legs. Pack some sandwiches and some easy-to-eat fruit such as apples, bananas or grapes. Some icy bottled water is also a good idea, especially during summer.

A self-catered holiday—in an apartment or holiday house—will give you far more control over your food choices, but, understandably, you won't want to spend all your time preparing food! So make it easy with a little forethought and preparation.

Meals to make anywhere

- Make a homemade pizza from Lebanese bread, spread with cheese and toppings
- Combine a can of tuna, chopped tomatoes and some antipasto vegetables for an easy pasta sauce
- Burritos can be made out of avocado, tortillas and a can of Mexican beans

Snacks to have on hand when you're away

- Fresh fruit—try some locally grown produce
- Unsalted nuts and dried fruit

- A low saturated-fat dip such as hummus or mashed avocado, scooped up with carrot sticks and celery
- Low-fat fruit yoghurts

Simple barbecue meals

- Try pieces of marinated lean steak or green king prawns
- Add some vegetables to the barbecue: mushrooms, halved tomatoes, sliced potato, corn on the cob (in its sheath), pineapple, capsicum and onions
- For dessert, try barbecued bananas in their skin (for a treat, add some chocolate hazelnut spread!)
- A prepared salad such as coleslaw or tabbouli can be purchased, or make your own combination of fresh salad vegetables and add the dressing just before serving

Plan a picnic

- Olives, marinated mushrooms, marinated capsicum and eggplant, semi-dried tomatoes and a homemade pasta salad
- Vegetable frittata, a handful of salad greens and tiny new potatoes with vinegar and mint
- Lean cold meats such as turkey breast, ham, silverside, pastrami or marinated chicken drumsticks
- Smoked trout or salmon, fresh oysters, prawns or Balmain bugs
- Tabbouli, hummus, pita bread and thin slices of tender roast lamb with a chickpea or lentil salad
- Fresh fruits such as grapes, sliced mango and strawberries
- A piece of nice cheese and fresh sourdough bread

- Cool mineral or soda water with a twist of lime or lemon

Day-trip survival kit

- Cold bottled water
- Fresh sandwiches with easy, simple fillings such as sliced cheese and pickle, ham and mustard and turkey breast with cranberry jelly
- Washed and dried fresh fruit such as small crisp apples or grapes

Survival tips to help you when you're eating out

- *Don't go ravenously hungry*—If you are planning a big night out, don't starve yourself through the day. All that does is reduce your metabolic rate. Eat a light breakfast and lunch and, before you go, have a quick snack—try a slice of grainy bread. This takes the edge off your appetite and you will be less likely to overeat.
- *Take an extra walk*—When you know you will be eating and drinking more than usual, take some extra exercise, preferably beforehand. If it is feasible, walk to the restaurant. At the very least, try not to park right outside the restaurant.
- *Before you order ask for water* and guzzle some down before your meal. It will begin filling your stomach.
- *Bypass the bread*
- *Remember 1,2,3*—**1** Low-GI smart carbs; **2** Vegetables or salad; **3** Protein—choose from meat, seafood, poultry or a vegetarian alternative such as tofu
- *Keep it simple*

- *Halve it*—order an entrée for your main course or specify entrée sizing. Alternatively,
- *Eat only half of everything on your plate*
- *Hold the fries*
- *Pace yourself*—Try ordering one course at a time and then see how you feel. This gives the receptors in your stomach time to send a satiety signal to your brain.
- *Save sauce for the side*
- *Take your time*—Relax and enjoy the food that is being prepared for you, not by you.
- *If you don't want it, leave it*
- *Be discerning with drinks*—Make water your first choice. Ask for some routinely whether you feel like it or not. Chances are you will drink it if it is in front of you. Go easy on the sugary drinks because they tend to bypass satiety mechanisms. Drink no more than one to three glasses of alcohol. Remember, alcohol has almost twice as many kilojoules as carbohydrate.
- *Spoons for two*—Go ahead and have a dessert, but why not share it with someone?
- *Walk it off*—After a restaurant meal, walk home or back to the office and climb the stairs rather than using the lift.

Finding the low-GI choice on the menu

Indian food

The traditional accompaniment for Indian dishes is steamed Basmati rice, which is a classic low-GI choice. Lentil dhal offers another low-GI accompaniment, but make sure they don't add the oil topping (tadka).

Unleavened breads such as chapatti or roti may have a lower GI than normal bread but it will boost the carbohydrate content of the meal and increase the glycemic load.

Our suggestions:
- Tikka (dry roasted) or tandoori (marinated in spices and yoghurt) chicken
- Basmati rice
- Cucumber raita
- Spicy spinach (saag)

Japanese food

Japanese sushi rice has a low GI, and any refrigerated rice has a lower GI than when it is freshly cooked. The vinegar used in preparation of sushi helps keep the GI low (acidity helps slow stomach emptying), and so do the viscous fibres in the seaweed. Typical ingredients and flavours to enjoy are shoyu (Japanese soy sauce), mirin (rice wine), wasabi (a strong horseradish), miso (soybean paste), pickled ginger (oshinko), sesame seeds and sesame oil. Go easy on deep-fried dishes such as tempura.

Japanese restaurants are great places to stock up on omega-3 fats, as dishes such as sushi and sashimi made with salmon and tuna contain high amounts of beneficial polyunsaturated fatty acids.

Our suggestions:
- Miso soup
- Sushi
- Teppanyaki (steak, seafood and vegetables)

- Yakitori (skewered chicken and onions in teriyaki sauce)
- Sashimi (thinly sliced raw fish or beef)
- Shabu-shabu (thin slices of beef quickly cooked with mushrooms, cabbage and other vegetables)
- Side orders such as seaweed salad, wasabi, soy sauce and pickled ginger

Thai food

Thai food is generally sweet and spicy and contains aromatic ingredients such as basil, lemongrass and galangal. Spicy Thai salads which usually contain seafood, chicken or meat are a delicious light meal. For starters, avoid the deep-fried items such as spring rolls.

One downside to Thai cuisine is the coconut milk, which really raises the saturated fat content of Thai curry. So don't feel you have to consume all of the sauce or soup. The traditional accompaniment to Thai food is plain, steamed Jasmine rice, but this is very high GI so you are better off if you can reduce the quantity. Noodles are always on the menu as well, but avoid fried versions. Boiled rice noodles may be an option. Limit yourself to a small helping or, if you are having takeaway, you could cook up some Doongara CleverRice at home as an accompaniment.

Our suggestions:
- Tom yam—hot and sour soup
- Thai beef or chicken salad
- Wok-tossed meats or seafood
- Stir-fried mixed vegetables
- Small serve of steamed noodles or rice
- Fresh spring rolls (not fried)

Italian food

The big plus with Italian restaurants is the supply of low-GI pasta with an array of sauces. Good choices are arrabiata, puttanesca, Napoletana and marinara sauces (without cream). Despite what you may think, most Italians don't sit down to huge bowls of pasta, so don't be afraid to leave some on your plate (or order an entrée size)—the GI may be low but a large serve of pasta will have a high GL. Other good choices include minestrone and vegetable dishes, lean veal and grilled seafood. Steer clear of crumbed and deep-fried seafood.

Our suggestions:

- Minestrone
- Veal escalopes in tomato-based sauce
- Prosciutto (paper-thin slices of smoky ham) wrapped around melon
- Barbecued or grilled seafood such as calamari or octopus
- Roasted or char-grilled fillet of beef, lamb loin or poultry
- Green garden salad with olive oil and balsamic vinegar
- Sorbet, gelato or simply a fresh fruit platter
- Entrée-size pasta with seafood and tomato or stock-based sauce

Greek and Middle Eastern food

In Mediterranean cuisine, olive oil, lemon, garlic and onions and other vegetables abound. Many dishes are char-grilled and specialities such as barbecued octopus or grilled sardines are excellent choices. You will find regular bread replaced with flat bread or Turkish bread, while potatoes are replaced with wholegrains such as bulgur (in tabbouli) and couscous.

Among the small appetising mezze dishes, you could pick and choose what you like. Many of the choices are healthy, such as hummus, baba ghanoush, olives, tzatziki and dolmades.

Our suggestions:

- Mezze platter with Lebanese bread
- Souvlaki (char-grilled skewers of meat with vegetables)
- Kofta (balls of minced lamb with bulgur wheat)
- Greek salad of fresh lettuce, tomato, olives, feta and capsicum, with balsamic dressing or oil and lemon
- Fresh fruit platter
- Felafel with tabbouli and hummus with a flat bread

Ten tips for people who regularly eat at restaurants

1 *Walk* to the restaurant if possible.
2 Order water as soon as you arrive.
3 Send the bread basket away (unless it's *exceptional*).
4 Order green salad, oysters au naturel or soup for entrée.
5 Order an entrée for your main course (or specify entrée size).
6 Alternatively, eat *only half* of everything on your plate.
7 Tell the waiter to hold the hot chips.
8 Share dessert with a dining companion.
9 Drink no more than one to three glasses of alcohol.
10 Walk back to the office or climb the stairs.

Staying on track while travelling for business

Breakfast

Good options include:

- Fruit—fruit or fresh juice is always available and this is a great way to boost your daily fruit intake. Try a fruit you've never had before with yoghurt on top.
- Cereal with low-fat milk—dry packet cereals need careful selection. Muesli, fruit and yoghurt is a more sustaining option.
- Cooked breakfast—go with the grainy bread for toast, skip the butter or margarine, and top it with poached or scrambled eggs. This gives you protein without too many kilojoules and can make everything more sustaining. Side orders such as mushrooms and tomato add micronutrients without excessive kilojoules.

Lunch

Lunch these days is mostly a light affair, but if it isn't, try to make your evening meal light. By light we mean big on salad and vegetables.

Dinner

Stick with simple options for dinner—grilled steak, chicken breast, fish or seafood with vegetables or salad. While ordering, think about how much energy you have used during the day, and order to match that.

Snacks

For a start, empty the mini bar and stock it with a couple of low-fat yoghurts and a few bananas or apples. Another solution is to prepare snacks in advance and take enough to last you through the trip. Dried fruit and nuts make lightweight, nutritious snacks.

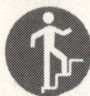

ACTIVITY TIP

While away on business, confined to hotel rooms and meeting rooms, it can be hard to find any time for activity. We suggest you pack a skipping rope and find 15 minutes a day to exercise in your hotel room. Alternatively, if the firestairs are accessible and safe, ask for a room on the second or third floor and use them as you come and go.

How to find a good dietitian

Dietitians have professionally recognised qualifications in human nutrition. They can provide specific advice tailored to your current eating habits and food preferences, and will work with you to set realistic and achievable goals. They will help you understand the relationship between food and health and guide you in making dietary choices that optimise your lifestyle. Dietitians practise as individual professionals and are available through most public hospitals and in private practice. To find a dietitian visit 'Find a Dietitian' at www.daa.asn.au or call 1800 812 942 in Australia or go to www.dietitians.org.nz in New Zealand.

What you need to do—activity and exercise

The single most important difference between long-term weight losers and weight gainers is the amount of physical activity they build into their day. Quite simply, exercise has to be your first priority. The aim in the 'Doing it for life' phase is to maintain the same activity level of Week 12 (see pages 176–78) but build in different forms of exercise so that you don't become bored. Setting new goals and enjoying what you do are critical.

Food minus exercise equals fat!

In short, building exercise into your life is vital. This does not mean you need to go and join the gym or start pounding the streets every night. There are lots of options, and finding what sort of exercise is suitable and enjoyable to you is the key to success.

Take five minutes every day to:	Potential saving in kilos of fat*	
	in 1 year	in 5 years
Take the stairs instead of the lift	3.7	18.5
Weed one patch of the garden	0.6	3.0
Rake the lawn	0.6	3.0
Vacuum the lounge room	0.7	3.5
Walk 150 m from the car to the office	0.7	3.5
Carry the groceries 150 m back to the car	0.9	4.5

*Figures are based on a 70 kg (11 stone) person.

This shows us that all those seemingly small actions where we *choose* to take the more active option really do add up in the long run. It won't hurt you to park your car at the furthest end of the car park. It might not feel as if climbing one flight of stairs makes a difference. But it does—you can save yourself 1 or 2 kilos of fat over the course of a year. Similarly, even if you have just five minutes rather than 30 minutes to fit in some exercise, do it anyway.

Types of exercise

While exercise works through three different systems, many forms of exercise work more than one system and sometimes all three. Cycling, for example, is primarily an aerobic exercise, but also involves resistance training for the legs as they have to push against a force. Yoga is usually thought of as primarily improving flexibility, yet holding the poses involves a good deal of resistance training using your body weight as resistance.

In your initial 12-week Weight-loss Plan we focused on aerobic exercise (walking) and resistance training in the

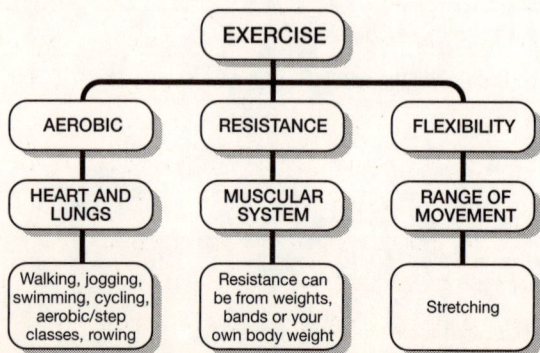

```
                    ┌─────────────┐
                    │  EXERCISE   │
                    └─────────────┘
        ┌──────────────────┼──────────────────┐
 ┌─────────────┐    ┌─────────────┐    ┌─────────────┐
 │   AEROBIC   │    │ RESISTANCE  │    │ FLEXIBILITY │
 └─────────────┘    └─────────────┘    └─────────────┘
 ┌─────────────┐    ┌─────────────┐    ┌─────────────┐
 │ HEART AND   │    │  MUSCULAR   │    │  RANGE OF   │
 │   LUNGS     │    │   SYSTEM    │    │  MOVEMENT   │
 └─────────────┘    └─────────────┘    └─────────────┘
 ┌─────────────┐    ┌─────────────┐    ┌─────────────┐
 │Walking,     │    │Resistance   │    │             │
 │jogging,     │    │can be from  │    │ Stretching  │
 │swimming,    │    │weights,     │    │             │
 │cycling,     │    │bands or your│    │             │
 │aerobic/step │    │own body     │    │             │
 │classes,     │    │weight       │    │             │
 │rowing       │    │             │    │             │
 └─────────────┘    └─────────────┘    └─────────────┘
```

form of key exercises you could do at home. Both these forms of exercise are most effective in helping you to lose body fat and they continue to be important from now on in assisting you to prevent a regain of weight. This doesn't mean that flexibility training is any less important—you should always stretch at the end of your exercise session—but spending more time on the types of exercise that will specifically help your weight control is just good time management. Let's take a look at some popular forms of exercise and see where they fit in with this model.

Walking and jogging

Walking is undoubtedly one of the best forms of exercise you can do for your health and almost anyone can do it. Continuing with your walking program may be all you want to do at this point and that is fine. If you are ready to step up your fitness a little more, you can raise the intensity, building up to a jog, or increase the time you spend walking.

Aerobics classes

Although these are primarily aerobic workouts many will also incorporate some resistance exercises and a good class will always include a stretch at the end. Group fitness classes are an excellent way to motivate you to exercise a little harder—the combination of uplifting music, guidance from a qualified instructor and the group atmosphere makes classes fun and effective. There are now classes to suit everyone—choose from aerobics, step, boxing, martial arts or circuit training. Classes are run in health clubs, leisure centres, universities and local halls all around the country.

Cycling

Cycling is primarily aerobic exercise but also involves some resistance training for the legs. Once you are geared up and ready to go, this is an excellent form of exercise to keep burning the kilojoules and preventing weight regain. Of course this needn't be a solo activity—try getting the whole family involved on the weekend or join a cycling group in your area for organised routes and social contact. The other option is to go along to an indoor group cycling class at your local health club. These are instructor led with motivating music to inspire you to give your best.

Rowing and kayaking

Rowing and kayaking mainly provide aerobic exercise, but since you are also using both upper and lower body strength you incorporate a good deal of resistance training at the same time.

Tennis, squash and other racket sports

These sports provide effective aerobic exercise, plus the social aspect helps you to keep it up. If you have never played before, book yourself in for a program of lessons.

Golf

While not as intense as some of the other forms of exercise, golf does take a long time to play and can be a great way to assist your weight loss. Of course, you need to walk to gain the benefits so leave the golf buggy at the clubhouse!

Weight training

The people who really need to weight train are not the young guns spotted pumping iron at your local gym, but the rest of us. As you already know, increasing your muscle mass raises your metabolic rate and helps you burn more fat all of the time, but did you know that weight training also strengthens your bones and can help to prevent weight gain as we age? This means that weight training is important for women approaching menopause, those at risk of osteoporosis, seniors and anyone who wants to control their weight. Health clubs now have sophisticated equipment that ensures you train effectively and safely—or you can work with resistance bands or join a weights-based group exercise class.

Team sports

If you enjoy the competition and camaraderie of team sports, then find a local team playing whatever sport you fancy. You could try soccer, netball, hockey, basketball, rugby or baseball. All these are great aerobic training and clubs often have a training program that also incorporates resistance and flexibility training.

Pilates and yoga

These classes focus more on flexibility but have a good element of resistance training—as you will know if you have ever tried to hold a yoga pose or taken part in a Pilates class. They have very little aerobic benefit, however, and, while they are a good addition to your exercise program, ensure that you also include some form of aerobic training.

Whatever type of exercise you decide on, the two important factors are that you enjoy the exercise and you do it regularly.

Swimming

Water provides 15 times more resistance than air. For this reason working out in water can be extremely effective. If you are very overweight or suffer from arthritis or other injury, getting in the water offers a safe and effective means of exercising. The water supports your body weight, your muscles work against the resistance of the water and you won't feel sore afterwards (muscle soreness comes mainly from muscles lengthening under resistance—in water the opposing muscle takes over so muscles only ever have to contract against the resistance). Choose from swimming laps or joining an aqua aerobics class in which an instructor will lead you through a series of exercises in the water.

Dancing

Dance classes are a fabulous way to get active and meet new friends. Choose from jazz, salsa, Scottish dancing, line dancing, ballet and ballroom—the choice is endless. See what appeals to you and what is available in your area.

Using a pedometer to achieve your steps or walking goal

A pedometer is highly effective in helping you achieve a walking goal. It counts the number of steps you take during the day, which can be a real eye-opener as to how active you really are! How many steps should you be taking?

- For optimum health: aim to achieve 7500 steps per day.
- For weight loss during the 12-week Weight-loss Plan: aim to achieve 10 000 steps per day.
- To prevent weight regain: aim to achieve 12 500 steps per day.

How to step up to these levels

- Wear your pedometer for the first week of 'Doing it for Life' and, at the end of each day, record the number of steps you took.
- Work out your average daily steps at the end of the week and add 30 per cent. This is your new goal for the next two to three weeks.
- Once you are achieving the new step goal easily, add a further 30 per cent. Repeat this process, taking as long as you need at each stage, until you are meeting the goals below.

The pedometer only counts the actual walking that you do and not other activities. The following table gives you an idea of how many steps are equivalent to 15 minutes of certain activities. Using these guidelines, you can reduce your daily step goal on days when you complete some other exercise or activity.

15 minutes of activity	Equivalent number of steps
Moderate sexual activity	500
Standing while watering lawn or garden	600
Vigorous sexual activity	750
Clearing and washing dishes	900
Standing while cooking at the barbecue	950
Standing while playing with kids	1100
Playing frisbee	1200
Ten-pin bowling	1200
Playing golf at the driving range	1200
Food shopping with a trolley	1400
General house cleaning	1400
Bicycling moderately (18 km/h)	1600
Raking the lawn	1600
Playing actively with kids	1600
Sweeping	1600
Horse riding	1600
Playing table tennis	1600
Washing the car by hand	1850
Spreading soil with a shovel	1950
Cleaning gutters of house	2000
Walk/run while playing vigorously with kids	2000
Digging or cultivating the garden	2000
Mowing the lawn with a hand mower	2350
Moving furniture	2350
Using heavy tools—e.g. shovel or crow bar	3150

What about joining a health club?

Health clubs are a great way to build exercise into your life—you have expert advice from qualified instructors, group fitness classes to choose from, a program designed for you in the gym and many also have a pool, squash courts or an associated running club.

Nevertheless your first visit can be a little daunting. Do your research first and find a club that meets your needs:

- Is it within a 15-minute drive from either your home or work?
- If you have young children, is there a crèche?
- What are the opening hours—if you want to go in the early morning or late evening are there classes at these times?
- If you think you would enjoy swimming or aqua classes, is there a pool?
- Will an instructor provide a gym program to get you started?
- What are the membership fee options and what is the get-out clause if you wish to cease membership?

What about a personal trainer?

There is no doubt that employing a personal trainer is a terrific way to improve your fitness and progress towards your goals. A good trainer will provide an individualised, progressive program as well as much needed motivation and support. Many personal trainers now provide services for a reasonable rate and you can choose to use a health club or train outdoors. A good way to bring the cost down is to train with a small group of three or four others with similar fitness levels.

How to find a good personal trainer

If you belong to a health club you should be able to find a personal trainer there. For working out in your own home or outdoors, look in your local newspaper or search online for someone in your area. Ask to see their qualifications—they should have a Certificate IV in training. Any good trainer will offer you at least one complimentary session to 'try before you buy'—to make sure you like the style of your trainer and can work well with him or her before you sign up for a number of sessions.

What if I don't have access to a personal trainer or health club, or can't afford it?

Use the 'buddy system'—you can get all the support and motivation you need from exercising with a buddy who has similar goals. Having an appointment to go walking or swimming with a friend makes it harder to be distracted or find an excuse to put it off. Remember, you are also offering the same motivation and support to your buddy so that you are both more likely to succeed.

Get the kids moving, too

Kids of active parents/guardians are far more likely to be active themselves—if not now, at least in the future. You may even persuade them to come exercising with you! Here are some tips:

1 Restrict periods of extended inactivity such as watching television or videos or playing computer games.

2 Invent projects to create at home (like a go-cart or a bird feeder).

3 Don't encourage sedentary behaviour over activity. (You may have to delete 'sit down and be quiet' from your vocabulary.)

4 Make sure the kids aren't watching you watching television.

5 Let them see you being active.

6 Don't chauffeur them, let them use public transport.

7 Don't confine them to the four walls of home or school.

8 Don't restrict spontaneous decisions to be active.

9 Put the ride-on toys and trampoline where they catch attention.

10 Prepare food with their help. They could help you with a special dish.

How much do you need to do?

Try to do something active on most days and add the following:

- Three cardiovascular sessions—this could be a group fitness class, cycling, a brisk walk or swimming.

- Two resistance workouts—either continue with your program from Week 12 (pages 176–78), or join a weights-based group fitness class, or have a program designed for you at your local health club. Yoga and Pilates classes will also improve your strength and muscletone, though to a lesser extent.

Twenty minutes of exercise gives you a mood boost and a natural high.

Tip: Put your exercise plans in your diary. Writing exactly what you are going to do in your diary and treating it as any other appointment, will help you stick to the plan.

What you need to know about using drugs to treat weight concerns

If you have done your best with a serious attempt at weight loss over three months, even with the additional help of a dietitian or personal trainer, and still feel dissatisfied with the amount of weight loss, we recommend a visit to your doctor. If you are markedly overweight—if your waist circumference is over 102 centimetres (male) or 88 centimetres (female)—he or she may refer you to an endocrinologist who specialises in obesity management. Apart from medication, there are surgical interventions to help those who are extremely overweight.

Looking forward to the one-year mark

A year of following a low-GI diet will give you a new lease of life. Having lost at least 5 to 10 per cent of your initial body weight, you will be fitting into clothes one or two sizes smaller, you will look and feel terrific and you will feel an undeniable buzz every time you have done your exercise for the day. Most importantly, you will have maintained the weight you lost and developed the confidence and know-how that ensures you keep it off for the rest of your life. Sure, there will be times when you gain a little, but that's normal and it shouldn't faze you, as you know you can repeat the Weight-loss Plan and shed the kilos at any stage. You will have learnt exactly what it takes to keep your weight under control through the recommendations in this chapter. It is not just about eating but also physical activity and balancing the energy equation. You have adopted a lifestyle, not a 'diet'.

The amount of weight you have lost may not take you back to your weight at age 18 or 25 but it doesn't matter. The weight you lose in this first year is what makes the world of difference to your health and wellbeing. While it might not be uppermost in your mind right now, living the healthy low-GI life will be giving you lots of value-added benefits, such as reducing the likelihood that you will develop

> Putting your health first gives you the best possible chance of achieving not only lifelong dreams, but everything else life puts on your plate.

diabetes, heart disease, arthritis, cancer and a number of other diseases. Your quality of life will remain high as the years advance, and you will be in the best shape possible to meet the challenges and pleasures of middle and older age.

Chapter 5
Low GI Diet Recipes

IN THIS SECTION YOU'LL FIND 50-PLUS RECIPES AND MEAL
ideas to help you put the GI to work in your kitchen—and
throughout your day. We have chosen recipes that will give
you a healthy balance of all the nutrients your body needs.

We have analysed the recipes, and the nutrient profile*
includes the GI, energy, fat, protein, carbohydrate and fibre
per serve. As discussed on page 44, in each recipe we have
noted the equivalent serve value of carbohydrate, protein,
fat and vegetables in each portion. This information is what
you need to follow the Low GI Diet 12-week Weight-loss
Plan and make it work for you.

GI: An emphasis on low-GI carbs such as pasta, legumes,
sweet potato, wholegrains, fruit and dairy ensures most of
our recipes have a low GI. The value we give is our best
estimate of the range in which the GI of each recipe falls.

---

* Recipes have been analysed using nutrient analysis software,
  FoodWorks® (Xyris Software), based on Australian and New Zealand
  food composition data

- Low GI 55 or below
- Medium or moderate GI 56–69
- High GI 70 or more

ENERGY DENSITY: The kilojoule count per serve of each recipe indicates its energy density. This is important to weight control because it's easy to overconsume kilojoules when your diet is based on energy-dense foods. By incorporating lots of vegetables, salads, fruits and high-fibre foods into recipes, they retain a lower energy density.

FATS: The type of fat is more important than the total amount. Most of us need to eat more of certain kinds of fats for optimal health. These fats include the omega-3 fats found in fish and seafood and omega-neutral monounsaturated fats found in olive and canola oils.

PROTEIN: Sufficient protein in the diet is important for weight control. Compared to carbohydrate and fat, protein makes us feel more satisfied immediately after eating and reduces hunger between meals. Protein also increases our metabolic rate for 1–3 hours after eating. This means we burn more energy by the minute compared with the increase that occurs after eating carbohydrates or fats. Even though this is a relatively small difference it may be important in long-term weight control.

CARBOHYDRATE: Many of our recipes have a carbohydrate base but the emphasis is always on low GI because the slow digestion and absorption of these foods will fill you up, trickle fuel into your engine at a more useable rate and keep you satisfied for longer. The actual amount of carbohydrate consumed at each meal may be relevant to those with diabetes and those who monitor their blood glucose levels.

FIBRE: Experts recommend a daily fibre intake of 30 grams, but most people fall short of that, averaging 20–25 grams. A low-GI diet will bring you a lot closer to the target because most of our recipes are brimming with fibre. This means they'll not only keep you regular but will help lower your blood glucose, your cholesterol levels and reduce your risk of many chronic diseases.

Breakfast, light meals and brunches

Breakfast on the Go

A quick and healthy breakfast drink.

Per serve
kJ/Cal 1500/353   **Protein** 27 g   **Fat** 4 g (saturated 1 g)
Carbohydrate 55 g   **Fibre** 3 g   **GI** Low

Preparation time 5 minutes
Cooking time nil   **Serves** 2

500 ml low-fat milk or soy beverage

½ cup low-fat natural yoghurt

½ punnet strawberries, hulled and chopped (optional)

1 large, ripe banana, roughly chopped

1 egg

1 tablespoon honey

1 tablespoon All-Bran® or wheat germ or psyllium husks

1 Combine the ingredients in a blender.

2 Process until smooth and frothy.

3 Pour into two glasses, drink and go!

Serves per portion
Protein 1.5   **Fruit** 1

Fruity Porridge Oats

You can make the dried fruit mixture in advance. Keep it in the refrigerator for 3–4 days and use as required. It can be served hot or cold on the porridge.

Per serve
kJ/Cal 1075/255   **Protein** 8 g   **Fat** 3 g (saturated <1 g)
Carbohydrate 48 g   **Fibre** 4 g   **GI** Low

Preparation time 5 minutes (plus soaking time)
Cooking time 20 minutes   **Serves** 4

100 g dried fruit (mixture of prunes, apricots, pears, apples, sultanas)
2 × 2.5 cm slices lemon rind
½ teaspoon cinnamon
2 cloves
300 ml unsweetened apple juice
125 g porridge oats
1½ cups (375 ml) low-fat milk

1 Place the dried fruit, lemon rind, cinnamon and cloves in a bowl. Pour over the apple juice, cover and leave in the refrigerator to soak overnight to bring out the flavours.

2 Transfer the ingredients to a heavy-based saucepan and bring to the boil, then reduce the heat and leave to simmer gently for about 15 minutes, stirring occasionally.

3 Put the oats in a saucepan with the milk and bring to the boil (making sure it doesn't boil over) then reduce the heat and simmer for 5 minutes.

4 Serve the porridge in small bowls topped with a spoonful or two of the dried fruit compote (warm or cold as preferred).

Serves per portion
Protein 0.5   **Carb** 1   **Fruit** 2

Egg and Bacon Tarts

*These tarts are delicious, simple and healthy to make for a cooked breakfast
or brunch. The high fat content makes them a weekend treat.*

Per serve
kJ/Cal 1640/386   **Protein** 28 g   **Fat** 18 g (saturated 6 g)
Carbohydrate 30 g   **Fibre** 4 g   **GI** Low

Preparation time 10 minutes
Cooking time 20–25 minutes   **Serves** 2

4 slices grainy bread
spray olive or canola oil
4 small eggs
2 rashers short-cut rindless bacon, trimmed of all fat and finely diced
¼ cup grated reduced-fat cheese
1 tablespoon parsley, chopped

1 Preheat the oven to 180°C.

2 Trim any thick or hard crusts from the bread and flatten each slice by rolling gently with a rolling pin.

3 Spray a medium-cup muffin pan with the oil and gently push each slice of bread into its own cup to line it. Spray again.

4 Break an egg into each cup—don't worry if it overflows a little. Top each with some bacon, cheese and parsley.

5 Bake for 20–25 minutes or until set.

Serves per portion
Protein 1   **Fat** ½   **Carb** 2

Vegetable Frittata

A lovely light lunch, this frittata is also great for picnics. It is a good source of folate and rich in beta-carotene. Offer fresh sourdough bread alongside.

Per serve (with salad)
kJ/Cal 790/190   **Protein** 12 g   **Fat** 9 g (saturated 3 g)
Carbohydrate 14 g   **Fibre** 4 g   **GI** Low

Preparation time 20 minutes
Cooking time 45 minutes   **Makes** 4 wedges

1 teaspoon olive oil
1 small onion, finely chopped
1 clove garlic, crushed
2 cups (300 g) grated sweet potato
2 zucchinis, grated
¼ cup basil leaves, shredded
⅓ cup grated reduced-fat cheese
salt and freshly ground black pepper, to taste
4 eggs, lightly beaten
150 g cherry tomatoes, halved

To serve
100 g mixed salad leaves
squeeze of lemon juice

1 Preheat the oven to 180°C. Lightly grease a 20 cm round cake tin and line the base with non-stick baking paper.

2 Heat the olive oil in a non-stick frypan and cook the onion and garlic for 4 minutes, or until soft. Add the sweet potato and zucchini and cook, stirring, for 3 minutes until softened slightly.

3 Transfer the vegetable mixture to a bowl and cool slightly. Mix in the basil and cheese, and season with salt and pepper. Stir to combine evenly. Fold in the eggs, and pour the mixture into the prepared tin. Smooth the surface.

4 Arrange the cherry tomatoes over the mixture, cut side up, and press in gently. Bake for 45 minutes, until set and golden. Leave in the tin until just cool enough to handle, then turn out and quickly invert right-side-up onto a plate.

5 Cut the frittata into wedges and serve with salad leaves, lightly dressed with lemon juice.

Serves per portion
Protein 1   **Carb** 1   **Veg** 2

Salmon and Dill Omelette with Tomato Salad

This omelette is a fantastic source of omega-3 fats, thanks to the salmon and eggs. Serve with salad and rye bread.

Per serve (with bread and salad)
kJ/Cal 3260/767   **Protein** 42 g   **Fat** 45 g (saturated 12 g)
Carbohydrate 47 g   **Fibre** 10 g   **GI** Low

Preparation time 15 minutes
Cooking time 5 minutes   **Serves** 2

4 eggs, at room temperature

2 tablespoons low-fat milk

1 tablespoon fresh dill, chopped

salt and freshly ground black pepper, to taste

2 teaspoons monounsaturated, salt-reduced margarine

30 g baby spinach leaves

100 g smoked salmon, cut into thin strips

¼ cup (25 g) grated parmesan

Tomato salad

200 g cherry or grape tomatoes, halved

100 g snowpea sprouts, ends trimmed

1 large Lebanese cucumber, cut into small chunks

2 tablespoons commercial fat free dressing

1 ripe avocado, thinly sliced

To Serve

4 slices rye bread

1 Whisk together the eggs, milk, dill, salt and pepper in a bowl.

2 Place 1 teaspoon margarine in each of two small non-stick frypans. (If you don't have 2 small frypans, make one large omelette to share.) Heat over a medium heat until the margarine starts to bubble. Pour the egg mixture evenly among the two pans and reduce the heat to low. Cook for 2 minutes or until the omelette is almost set.

3 Place half the spinach, salmon and parmesan on one side of each omelette. Carefully fold the other side of the omelette over the filling.

4 Meanwhile, to make the salad, place the tomatoes, snowpea sprouts and cucumber in a bowl. Add the dressing and toss gently to combine. Add the avocado.

5 Serve the omelettes with the salad and bread.

Serves per portion
Protein 2   **Carb** 2   **Fat** 2   **Veg** 3

Ham, Corn and Zucchini Muffins

*Best eaten the day they are made, these muffins
are an excellent source of fibre.*

Per muffin	**Per serve (with salad)**
kJ/Cal 1314/309 **Protein** 15 g	**kJ/Cal** 1480/34 **Protein** 16 g
Fat 4 g (saturated 1 g) **Carbohydrate** 51 g	**Fat** 7 g (saturated 2 g) **Carbohydrate** 53 g
Fibre 6 g **GI** Medium	**Fibre** 7 g **GI** Medium

Preparation time 20 minutes
Cooking time 20 minutes   **Makes** 6 muffins

1 cup (150 g) self-raising flour
1 cup (160 g) wholemeal self-raising flour
1 teaspoon baking powder
2 tablespoons caster sugar
1 × 310 g can corn kernels, drained
1 zucchini (about 125 g), coarsely grated
100 g lean leg ham, finely chopped
⅓ cup (30 g) grated parmesan
¼ cup fresh chives, chopped
2 eggs
⅔ cup (160 ml) low-fat milk
½ cup (125 g) low-fat natural yoghurt

To serve

100 g mixed salad leaves or mesclun
1 red capsicum, cut into short, thin strips
100 g snowpeas, cut into long, thin strips
2 tablespoons vinaigrette

1 Preheat the oven to 200°C and lightly grease a 6 × 1 cup (250 ml) muffin pan.

2 Sift the flours and baking powder into a large bowl. Stir in the sugar, corn, zucchini, ham, parmesan and chives.

3 Whisk the eggs, milk and yoghurt together. Add to the dry ingredients and use a large metal spoon to mix until just combined. Spoon the mixture evenly among the greased pans. Bake for 20 minutes or until light golden brown on top and a skewer inserted in the centre comes out clean.

4 Meanwhile, combine the salad ingredients. Serve with the warm muffins.

Serves per portion
Protein ½   **Carb** 3   **Veg** ½ (or 2 with salad)

Fried Rice

The rice for this dish can be cooked and cooled a day ahead. Store in an airtight container in the refrigerator.

Per serve
kJ/Cal 1930/460   **Protein** 32 g   **Fat** 11.3 g (saturated 3 g)
Carbohydrate 55 g   **Fibre** 4 g   **GI** Low

Preparation time 15 minutes (plus cooling time)
Cooking time 25 minutes   **Serves** 4

1¼ cups (250 g) Basmati rice
1 tablespoon olive oil
3 eggs, at room temperature
1 red capsicum, finely chopped
250 g small cooked, peeled prawns
120 g leg ham, chopped
1 cup (155 g) frozen peas
4 shallots, thinly diagonally sliced
1 cup bean sprouts
2 tablespoons salt-reduced soy sauce

1   Cook the rice in a large saucepan of boiling water for 10–12 minutes or until tender. Drain well. Spread out in a single layer over two baking trays. Set aside to cool completely.

2   Heat half the oil in a large non-stick wok or frypan over a medium heat. Whisk the eggs until frothy. Pour into the wok or pan and swirl to cover the base. Cook for 2 minutes or until the egg is set. Carefully loosen the edges and turn out onto a board. Set aside to cool. Roll up the omelette and cut into thin strips. Set aside.

3   Heat the remaining oil in the wok over a high heat. Add the capsicum, prawns, ham and peas. Cook, tossing, for 2 minutes. Add the shallots and toss for 1 minute. Add the cooled rice and toss until heated through. Add the bean sprouts and soy sauce. Toss to combine and serve.

Serves per portion
Protein 2   **Fat** ½   **Carb** 3   **Veg** 1

Ham and Vegetable Bake

This is a terrific recipe for kids—both to make and eat! It is an easy dish that can be eaten hot, warm or cold, and it is great for picnics, too.

Per serve
kJ/Cal 1240/292   **Protein** 18 g   **Fat** 10 g (saturated 4 g)
Carbohydrate 30 g   **Fibre** 6 g   **GI** Low

Preparation time 10 minutes
Cooking time 40 minutes   **Serves** 6

4 eggs
1 × 400 g can salt reduced corn kernels, drained
2 slices (50 g) leg ham, diced
½ cup grated reduced-fat tasty cheese
2 zucchinis, grated
2 carrots, grated
1 onion, grated
½ cup (160 g) wholemeal self-raising flour

1 Preheat the oven to 150°C and grease a large lasagne dish.

2 Lightly whisk the eggs in a large mixing bowl. Add the corn, ham, cheese, zucchini, carrot and onion, then sift in the flour and mix thoroughly to combine.

3 Spoon the mixture into the lasagne dish and press down to flatten the top. Bake for 40 minutes until browned and set.

Serves per portion
Protein 1   **Fat** ½   **Carb** 2   **Veg** 1

Turkey and Peach Salsa Wraps

Rich in protein and low in fat, these wraps make a delicious and nutritious lunch. Use canned peaches when fresh peaches are not in season—just make sure they are well drained.

Per wrap
kJ/Cal 959/226   **Protein** 25 g   **Fat** 4 g (saturated 1 g)
Carbohydrate 21 g   **Fibre** 4 g   **GI** Medium

Preparation time 15 minutes
Cooking time nil   **Makes** 2 wraps

1 peach, peeled and chopped
½ Lebanese cucumber, chopped
2 teaspoons mint, chopped
1 shallot, sliced
30 g iceberg lettuce leaves
2 sheets wholemeal lavash bread
150 g turkey slices

1 Combine the peach, cucumber, mint and shallots.

2 Spread the lettuce leaves over two-thirds of the lavash bread. Arrange the turkey slices over the lettuce.

3 Spoon the peach salsa over the turkey. Roll up to enclose the filling. If not serving immediately, wrap in paper or foil and store for up to 5 hours. Keep cool.

Serves per portion
Protein 1½   **Carb** 1   **Veg** 1

Tuna Rice Paper Rolls

If you like, use mint instead of coriander in these Vietnamese-style rolls, or leave it out altogether. Plain soy sauce makes a quick dipping sauce if you don't have the other ingredients. A good source of omega-3 fats, these rolls are also high in protein and rich in beta-carotene and vitamin C.

Per serve (3 rolls)
kJ/Cal 680/160   **Protein** 24 g   **Fat** 3 g (saturated 1 g)
Carbohydrate 8 g   **Fibre** 3 g   **GI** Medium

Preparation time 30 minutes
Cooking time nil   **Makes** 12 rolls

12 × 23 cm round rice paper sheets

1 × 425 g can tuna in spring water, drained and flaked

1 carrot, grated

2 shallots, finely sliced

2 cups (200 g) mung bean sprouts

½ cup (15 g) coriander leaves

1 red capsicum, finely sliced

Dipping sauce
1 tablespoon fish sauce
2 tablespoons lime juice
1 tablespoon sweet chilli sauce

1 Pour about 3 cm of tepid water into a large shallow dish. Dip one rice paper sheet in the water and soak for about 5 seconds, until just soft and pliable.

2 Drain and pat dry with paper towel. Place some of the tuna, carrot, shallots, sprouts, coriander and capsicum across one end of the sheet. Fold the end over, then the sides in. Roll up to enclose the filling securely. Repeat with the remaining rice paper sheets and filling ingredients.

3 Combine the fish sauce, lime juice and sweet chilli sauce. Serve in a small bowl for dipping.

Serves per portion
Protein 1½   **Carb** ½   **Veg** 2

Sweet Potato Fish Cakes

Per serve (2 fish cakes with salad)
kJ/Cal 911/214   **Protein** 21 g   **Fat** 4 g (saturated <1 g)
Carbohydrate 22 g   **Fibre** 5 g   **GI** Medium

Preparation time 20 minutes (plus chilling time)
Cooking time 15–20 minutes   **Makes** 12 fish cakes

750 g sweet potato, peeled and cut into 2 cm pieces

500 g boneless white fish fillets

2 teaspoons olive oil

1 leek, finely chopped

1 red capsicum, finely chopped

2 garlic cloves, crushed

2 tablespoons fresh parsley, chopped

salt and freshly ground black pepper, to taste

spray olive oil

To serve

100 g mixed salad leaves or mesclun

1 Lebanese cucumber, cut into chunks

2 ripe tomatoes, cut into chunks

2 tablespoons commercial fat free dressing

1 Steam or microwave the sweet potato until tender. Meanwhile, line a steamer basket with non-stick baking paper. Place the steamer basket over a wok or pan of just simmering water (make sure the water doesn't touch the basket), cover, and steam the fish for 5–10 minutes until cooked.

2 Heat the oil in a non-stick frypan over a medium heat. Add the leek, capsicum and garlic and cook, stirring often, for 6–7 minutes or until the leek is soft. Set aside.

3 Place the sweet potato in a bowl and mash until smooth. Use a fork to flake the fish into very small pieces. Add the leek mixture, fish and parsley to the sweet potato and stir well to combine. Season with salt and pepper. Cover and refrigerate until well chilled.

4 Shape the mixture into 12 patties. Place on two baking trays lined with non-stick baking paper. Refrigerate for 30 minutes. Preheat the oven to 200°C.

5 Spray both sides of the fish cakes lightly with oil. Bake for 15–20 minutes or until warmed through and light golden. Combine the salad ingredients and serve with the fish cakes.

Serves per portion
Protein 1½   **Carb** 1   **Veg** 2½

Indian Chicken Burgers

If you like, replace the tikka masala paste with any of your favourite Indian-style pastes. The cooked chicken patties are ideal to take on picnics or to work.

Per serve (patty)	Per serve (burger)
kJ/Cal 940/221 **Protein** 23 g	**kJ/Cal** 1920/460 **Protein** 32 g
Fat 10 g (saturated 2 g) **Carbohydrate** 10 g	**Fat** 12 g (saturated 2 g) **Carbohydrate** 52 g
Fibre 4 **GI** Low	**Fibre** 8 g **GI** Medium

Preparation time 20 minutes
Cooking time 10 minutes   **Makes** 6

500 g chicken breast fillets, chopped

1 bunch coriander, leaves picked

1 × 400 g can chickpeas, rinsed and drained

1 garlic clove, chopped

2 tablespoons tikka masala paste

2 teaspoons olive oil

To serve

1 × 430 g packet (45 cm long) Turkish bread, cut into 6 portions

100 g salad mix

3 small tomatoes, thinly sliced

½ cup (125 g) low-fat natural yoghurt

4½ tablespoons mango chutney

1 Place the chicken, coriander, chickpeas, garlic and tikka masala paste in a food processor. Process until the mixture is finely chopped and well combined. Shape the mixture into 6 patties. Refrigerate until required.

2 Heat the oil in a large non-stick frypan over a medium heat. Add the chicken patties and cook for 4–5 minutes on each side or until cooked through and light golden. Meanwhile, split and toast the Turkish bread portions.

3 Top the bases of the Turkish bread with the salad mix and tomatoes, then add a chicken patty each. Spoon over the yoghurt and chutney. Then add the tops of the Turkish bread and serve.

Serves per portion
Protein 2 **Fat** 1 **Carb** 3½ **Veg** 1

Lentil, Beetroot and Feta Salad

Per serve (salad only)
kJ/Cal 665/156   **Protein** 12 g
Fat 5 g (saturated <1 g)   **Carbohydrate** 12 g   **Fibre** 5 g   **GI** Low

Per serve (with bread)
kJ/Cal 1120/264   **Protein** 16 g   **Fat** 6 g (saturated 1 g)
Carbohydrate 32 g   **Fibre** 7 g   **GI** Low

Preparation time 15 minutes
Cooking time nil   **Serves** 4

1 × 400 g can brown lentils, rinsed and drained

100 g reduced-fat feta, cubed

125 g baby spinach leaves

1½ tablespoons lemon juice

1 teaspoon extra-virgin olive oil

1 teaspoon honey

1 cup (180 g) canned baby beets, drained and quartered

salt and freshly ground black pepper, to taste

4 thick slices sourdough rye bread

1 Combine the lentils, feta and spinach in a large bowl.

2 Place the lemon juice, oil and honey in a screwtop jar, and shake until well combined.

3 Drizzle the dressing over the lentil mixture and turn gently to coat.

4 Arrange the lentil mixture on serving plates, and add the beets. Season with salt and pepper, and serve immediately with the bread.

Serves per portion
Protein 1   **Fat** ½   **Carb** 1 (2 with bread)   **Veg** 1½

Thai-style Tofu and Noodle Soup

An excellent source of folate and vitamin C and a good source of calcium, magnesium and potassium, this soup is a meal in itself. The tofu doesn't need cooking, but adding it in at the beginning helps it to absorb the flavours. Lemongrass is available either fresh or in jars, from large supermarkets. Choose fresh if you can—for the best flavour. Mung bean vermicelli, sometimes called cellophane noodles or bean thread vermicelli, is available in the Asian food section of supermarkets.

Per serve
kJ/Cal 935/220   **Protein** 16 g   **Fat** 7 g (saturated 1 g)
Carbohydrate 21 g   **Fibre** 7 g   **GI** Low

Preparation time 20 minutes
Cooking time about 5 minutes   **Serves** 4

100 g mung bean vermicelli

4 cups (1 L) vegetable stock

1 tablespoon finely chopped lemongrass

1½ teaspoons finely grated ginger

1½ teaspoons finely chopped red chilli

350 g firm tofu, cut into 1.5 cm cubes

1 bunch asparagus, cut into 5 cm lengths

1 small head broccoli (about 300 g), cut into small florets

125 g baby corn, cut in half lengthways and crossways

2 shallots, finely sliced

fresh coriander leaves, to serve

1   Place the vermicelli in a large heatproof bowl and cover with boiling water. Leave to stand for 10 minutes.

2   Meanwhile, pour the vegetable stock into a large saucepan. Add the lemongrass, ginger, chilli and tofu. Bring to the boil.

3   Add the asparagus, broccoli and corn. Return to the boil, then cook for 2 minutes.

4   Drain the noodles then divide between four serving bowls and top with the vegetables, tofu and stock. Sprinkle each bowl with shallots and coriander leaves and serve immediately.

Serves per portion
Protein 1   **Carb** 1   **Veg** 2

Mains

Pasta with Char-grilled Chicken, Lemon and Basil

Per serve
kJ/Cal 2100/494   **Protein** 30 g   **Fat** 10 g (saturated 2 g)
Carbohydrate 70 g   **Fibre** 7 g   **GI** Low

Preparation time 15 minutes
Cooking time about 10 minutes   **Serves** 4

2 chicken breast fillets
spray olive oil
300 g short pasta, such as penne or spirals
1 cup (150 g) fresh or frozen green peas
300 g can corn kernels, well drained
1 tablespoon extra-virgin olive oil
2 tablespoons lemon juice
salt and freshly ground black pepper, to taste
½ cup basil leaves, shredded

1 Spray the chicken breast fillets lightly with oil and cook on a preheated char-grill or frypan for 5 minutes on each side, or until cooked through. Cool the chicken slightly, then slice thinly across the grain.

2 Meanwhile, cook the pasta in a large saucepan of boiling salted water according to packet directions, or until al dente. Add the peas and corn to the pasta for the last minute of cooking.

3 Drain the pasta, peas and corn, then return to the pan. Drizzle with the extra-virgin olive oil and lemon juice, and add the chicken. Season well with salt and pepper then toss to combine.

4 Spoon onto serving plates and top with the basil leaves. Serve immediately.

Serves per portion
Protein 2   **Carb** 4   **Fat** ½   **Veg** ½

Chicken Stuffed with Spinach and Cheese

This meal is high in folate, niacin, beta-carotene and fibre.

Per serve
kJ/Cal 2117/498   **Protein** 55 g   **Fat** 18 g (saturated 6 g)
Carbohydrate 26 g   **Fibre** 10 g   **GI** Low

Preparation time 15 minutes
Cooking time 25–30 minutes   **Serves** 4

4 chicken breast fillets (about 200 g each)

4 slices reduced-fat Swiss cheese (15 g each), cut into thin strips

80 g mushrooms, thinly sliced

40 g baby spinach leaves

4 wooden toothpicks

2 teaspoons olive oil

salt and freshly ground black pepper, to taste

1⅓ cups (330 ml) Italian tomato cooking sauce

⅓ cup fresh basil leaves, finely shredded

To serve
1 bunch baby carrots, washed
240 g green beans, trimmed
2 cobs fresh sweetcorn, halved

1   Preheat the oven to 180°C. Cut a deep slit (making sure not to cut all the way through) along the length of each chicken breast. Fill each evenly with the cheese, mushrooms and spinach. Secure the opening with toothpicks.

2   Heat the oil in a large non-stick frypan over a medium–high heat. Season both sides of the chicken breasts with salt and pepper. Cook for 2–3 minutes on each side or until well browned.

3   Transfer the chicken to a shallow ovenproof dish and pour over the cooking sauce. Bake for 15–20 minutes or until the chicken is cooked through.

4   Meanwhile, steam the carrots, beans and sweetcorn.

5   Remove the toothpicks and place the chicken breasts on serving plates. Pour over the sauce and sprinkle with the basil. Serve with the vegetables.

Serves per portion
Protein 4   **Fat** 1   **Carb** 1   **Veg** 3

Chicken and Rice Salad

This tasty meal is a good source of magnesium, niacin, vitamin C and vitamin A. Before serving, try scattering over some toasted cashew nuts.

Per serve
kJ/Cal 1326/312   **Protein** 21 g   **Fat** 5 g (saturated 1 g)
Carbohydrate 45 g   **Fibre** 2 g   **GI** Medium

Preparation time 20 minutes
Cooking time 12 minutes   **Serves** 4

2 (300 g) chicken breast fillets
1 cup (200 g) Basmati rice
1 tablespoon soy sauce
¼ teaspoon sesame oil
1 red capsicum, cut into thin strips
100 g snowpeas, sliced diagonally
1 carrot, grated
2 shallots, sliced diagonally
2 tablespoons lemon juice

1 Gently simmer the chicken in a saucepan of boiling water for 12 minutes, until tender. Remove from the pan. When cool enough to handle, cut into thin strips.

2 Meanwhile, cook the rice in a large saucepan of boiling water for about 10 minutes, until tender. Drain, rinse under cold water to stop the cooking, then drain completely.

3 Place the chicken on a plate. Combine the soy sauce and sesame oil and drizzle over the chicken. Toss to coat.

4 Combine the rice and vegetables in a large bowl. Drizzle over the lemon juice and toss to combine. Add the chicken to the rice, and mix through gently. Serve immediately, or refrigerate until serving time.

Serves per portion
Protein 1   **Carb** 2   **Veg** 1

Chinese Combination Soup for One

You can buy boiled wontons, lean barbecue pork and Chinese chicken stock in Chinese markets and Asian produce stores. Frozen wontons are also available in larger supermarkets. In this recipe, you can use any other Asian greens or vegetables such as handful of raw bean sprouts, baby corn or champignon mushrooms instead of the choy sum if you prefer. For a seafood combination soup use 2 or 3 prawns, 2 or 3 diced white fish cubes and 2 or 3 small pieces of squid instead of the pork and add a seafood stock.

Per serve
kJ/Cal 1860/445 **Protein** 36 g **Fat** 10 g (saturated 4 g)
Carbohydrate 50 g **Fibre** 4 g **GI** Low

Preparation time: 10 minutes

4 boiled wontons

40 g (small handful) egg noodles, blanched and drained

½ bunch choy sum, washed, leaves separated and blanched

6 slices of lean barbecue pork

2 cups (500 ml) hot Chinese chicken stock (or regular chicken stock)

To serve

1 tablespoon finely chopped shallots

1 tablespoon chopped fresh coriander

½ teaspoon finely chopped red chilli (optional)

1 Place the wontons, egg noodles, choy sum and pork in a single-serve large Chinese bowl. Ladle the stock over. Garnish with shallots and coriander and chilli if desired.

Serves per portion
Protein 2 **Carb** 3 **Veg** 2

Tandoori Chicken with Cumin-flavoured Rice

You can make this using a whole chicken as we have here or with chicken pieces if you prefer to reduce the cooking time.

Per serve (with cumin-flavoured rice)
kJ/Cal 2120/505   **Protein** 45 g   **Fat** 16 g (saturated 4 g)
Carbohydrate 44 g   **Fibre** 1 g   **GI** Low

Preparation time 20 minutes (plus 6–8 hours for marinating)
Cooking time about 50 minutes   **Serves** 4

1 medium chicken (about 800 g), cleaned and skin removed
1 teaspoon chilli powder
2 teaspoons lemon juice
salt to taste
3 teaspoons margarine

Marinade
250 ml low-fat plain yoghurt
1 teaspoon garam masala
1 teaspoon ground cumin
2 small red chillies, finely chopped (or to taste)
3 teaspoons finely grated ginger
3 teaspoons finely diced garlic
1 teaspoon lemon juice

To serve
3–4 tablespoons chopped coriander leaves
1 onion, finely sliced into rings
1 lemon cut into wedges

1 To prepare the chicken, combine the chilli powder, lemon juice and salt in a small bowl. Place the chicken in a shallow glass or ceramic dish. Using a sharp knife, make incisions on breast and leg pieces of the chicken. Rub the chilli mixture over the chicken, cover and set aside.

2 To make the marinade, combine the yoghurt in a bowl with the rest of the marinade ingredients and stir until thoroughly combined. Spoon the marinade mix all over the chicken, pushing it into the slits. Cover and place the chicken in the refrigerator for 6–8 hours to marinate. Turn occasionally to make sure all sides are coated in the mixture.

3 Preheat the oven to 200°C. Place the chicken on a wire rack over a large baking dish and roast for about 40–50 minutes, or until the chicken is cooked—the juices will run clear when you insert a skewer. Alternatively, skewer the chicken and cook it in a hot clay oven (tandoor) or barbecue it on an open hot grill. When the chicken is almost cooked, baste with melted margarine and roast for another 3 minutes.

4 While the chicken is cooking, prepare the cumin-flavoured rice (see below).

5 Serve with onion rings, chopped coriander, lemon wedges and cumin-flavoured rice.

Cumin-flavoured Rice

1 cup (200 g) Basmati rice
1½ cups (375 ml) water
1 teaspoon canola oil
2 teaspoons cumin seeds

1 Wash the rice well then place in a bowl, cover with cold water and soak for 30 minutes. Drain.

2 Heat the oil in a heavy-based pan, add the cumin and let it 'sputter' until aromatic. Add the rice and water, stir and bring to the boil. Reduce the heat to very low, cover the pan and cook for about 15–20 minutes or until all the water has evaporated.

Serves per portion
Protein 4 **Carb** 2 **Fat** 0.5

Eggplant and Zucchini Pilaf with Lamb

Per serve
kJ/Cal 2110/496   **Protein** 30 g   **Fat** 10 g (saturated 3 g)
Carbohydrate 70 g   **Fibre** 7 g   **GI** Medium

Preparation time 15 minutes
Cooking time 30 minutes   **Serves** 4

2 large red capsicums (about 200 g each), cut into 2.5 cm pieces

1 eggplant (about 300 g), cut into 2.5 cm pieces

2 large zucchinis (about 350 g each), cut into 2.5 cm pieces

4 teaspoons olive oil

salt and freshly ground black pepper, to taste

1 brown onion, finely chopped

2 garlic cloves, crushed

1½ cups (300 g) Basmati rice, rinsed

2½ cups (625 ml) salt-reduced chicken stock

2 lamb backstraps (about 200 g each)

1½ tablespoons fresh parsley, finely chopped

1 Preheat the oven to 230°C and line a large roasting pan with non-stick baking paper.

2 Place the capsicum, eggplant, zucchini and 2 teaspoons of oil in a bowl. Season with salt and pepper and toss well to coat. Spread in a single layer over the lined pan. Bake for 25–30 minutes or until very tender and light golden brown.

3 Meanwhile, heat 1 teaspoon of oil in a large, non-stick, heavy-based saucepan over a medium heat. Add the onion and garlic and cook, stirring often, for 7–8 minutes or until the onion is soft. Increase the heat to high and add the rice. Cook, stirring, for 1 minute. Add the stock, cover, and bring to the boil. Reduce the heat to low and cook, covered, for 10 minutes. Remove from the heat and set aside, covered, for 10 minutes.

4 Brush the lamb with the remaining oil and season with salt and pepper. Preheat a char-grill pan or frypan over a medium–high heat. Add the lamb and cook for 3–4 minutes on each side for medium, or until cooked to your liking. Set aside for 5 minutes, then slice diagonally.

5 Use a fork to fluff up the rice and separate the grains. Add the roasted vegetables and the parsley to the rice and toss gently to combine.

6 Divide the rice among serving plates and top with the lamb.

Serves per portion
Protein 4   **Carb** 4   **Fat** ½   **Veg** 3

Barbecued Lamb with Lentil Salad and Lemon Yoghurt Dressing

Per serve
kJ/Cal 1900/447   **Protein** 49 g   **Fat** 16 g (saturated 4 g)
Carbohydrate 21 g   **Fibre** 11 g   **GI** Low

Preparation time 10 minutes (plus marinating time)
Cooking time 15 minutes   **Serves** 2

1 tablespoon olive oil
1 clove garlic, crushed
a few sprigs of fresh oregano, roughly torn
zest of 1 lemon
300–400 g lamb fillet or backstrap

Dressing
juice of 1 lemon
½ cup low-fat natural yoghurt
salt and freshly ground pepper, to taste

Salad
1 tablespoon olive oil
1 × 400 g can brown lentils, drained
2 medium tomatoes, diced
35 g baby spinach leaves, shredded

1 Combine the olive oil, garlic, oregano and lemon zest in a bowl. Add the lamb fillets or backstrap and marinate for at least 30 minutes. Brown the marinated lamb in a frypan over medium–high heat or on the barbecue until just cooked. Remove, cover and set aside.

2 Meanwhile, combine the lemon juice with the yoghurt in a small jar, leaving aside a squeeze of the lemon juice. Season with salt and pepper. Put on the lid and shake to combine.

3 To make the salad, heat the olive oil in a frypan over a medium heat and add the lentils, stirring to warm through. Add the tomatoes and spinach and a squeeze of lemon juice, and stir to combine. Remove from the heat.

4 Slice the lamb across the grain (about 1.5 cm thick).

5 Spoon the lentil salad onto serving plates. Top with the sliced meat and pour over the dressing.

Serves per portion
Protein 4   **Carb** 1   **Fat** 1   **Veg** 1½

Beef Kebabs with Vegetable Noodle Salad

Not only is this dish an excellent source of iron and zinc, it also contains vitamin C to enhance absorption of these nutrients. If time permits, you can marinate the meat on skewers overnight.

Per serve
kJ/Cal 1735/408   **Protein** 36 g   **Fat** 7 g (saturated 3 g)
Carbohydrate 50 g   **Fibre** 4 g   **GI** Low

Preparation time 20 minutes (plus marinating time)
Cooking time 10–15 minutes   **Serves** 4

500 g lean rump steak, cut across the grain into thin strips

16 wooden skewers, soaked in cold water for 15–20 minutes

⅓ cup (80 ml) plum sauce marinade

1 × 450 g packet Hokkien noodles

1 red capsicum, cut into short, thin strips

100 g snowpeas, cut into thin strips

1 Lebanese cucumber, cut into thin strips

1 bunch coriander, leaves picked

¼ cup (60 ml) salt-reduced soy sauce

¼ cup (60 ml) fat free French dressing

1 Thread the beef strips evenly among the skewers, then place the skewers in a shallow glass or ceramic dish. Pour over the marinade and turn to coat. Set aside for 1 hour to marinate.

2 Preheat a barbecue char-grill or frypan over a medium heat. Place the noodles in a large heatproof bowl and cover with boiling water. Set aside for 5 minutes. Drain well, set aside to cool slightly, then separate the noodles. Add the capsicum, snowpeas, cucumber and coriander, and toss to combine.

3 Whisk the soy sauce and dressing together. Add to the salad and toss to combine.

4 Cook the beef skewers for 2–3 minutes on each side or until cooked through. Serve with the noodle salad.

Serves per portion
Protein 3   **Carb** 3   **Veg** 1½

Mediterranean Beef Stew

Per serve
kJ/Cal 1280/305   **Protein** 35 g   **Fat** 12 g (saturated 4 g)
Carbohydrate 8 g   **Fibre** 4 g   **GI** Low

Preparation time 30 minutes
Cooking time about 2 hours   **Serves** 4

1 tablespoon olive oil

600 g trimmed beef suitable for a casserole, cut into 2.5 cm cubes

2 large onions, thinly sliced

1 clove garlic, crushed

½ cup red wine

1 cup Italian peeled tomatoes

1 large bay leaf

freshly ground black pepper, to taste

½ cup dried porcini mushrooms, rehydrated in ½ cup warm water

12 baby carrots, scrubbed and tops trimmed

1 teaspoon fresh thyme, finely chopped

1½ tablespoons fresh parsley, finely chopped

1 Preheat the oven to 180ºC

2 Heat the oil in a large flameproof casserole dish then brown the cubes of beef on all sides, cooking a few at a time. Transfer the browned meat to a plate and set aside.

3 Reduce the heat then add the onions and cook for 3 or 4 minutes until they are soft and golden. Stir in the crushed garlic and add the meat cubes.

4 Add the wine, tomatoes and the bay leaf and season with freshly ground black pepper to taste. Bring to a simmer then cover with a tightly fitting lid, transfer to the middle shelf of the oven and cook for 1 hour.

5 Remove from the oven and stir in the mushrooms, the water they have been soaking in, the carrots and herbs and mix well. Return to the oven and cook for a further 30 minutes or until the carrots are soft.

6 Serve over noodles or Basmati rice with a salad or green vegetables.

Serves per portion
Protein 4   **Fat** 0.5   **Veg** 2

Claypot Rice with Minced Pork, Eggplant and Spinach

For this recipe you need a 2-person claypot (1.25 litre capacity).
If you don't have a claypot, use a cast-iron enamel pot.

Per serve
kJ/Cal 2155/515   **Protein** 31 g   **Fat** 18 g (saturated 4 g)
Carbohydrate 51 g   **Fibre** 10 g   **GI** Medium

Preparation time 15 minutes
Cooking time 15 minutes   **Serves** 2

spray olive oil

2 cups freshly steamed Basmati or Doongara CleverRice (made with 100 g uncooked rice)

1 bunch Chinese water spinach or English spinach, chopped and stir-fried

1 tablespoon olive oil

300 g baby eggplant, sliced

200 g minced pork

1 tablespoon finely chopped garlic

1 tablespoon finely chopped fresh ginger

2 tablespoons finely chopped shallots

1 tablespoon dark soy sauce

1 tablespoon rice wine

1 tablespoon Chinese black rice vinegar

2 teaspoons sugar

1 teaspoon Sichuan peppercorns, roasted and crushed

1 teaspoon chilli powder

50 ml (2½ tablespoons) Chinese chicken stock or water

1 Prepare the claypot by spraying thoroughly inside with olive oil.

2 To prepare the minced pork and eggplant, heat a wok and add the olive oil. Stir-fry the sliced eggplant till soft. Add the pork, garlic, ginger, shallots, soy sauce, rice wine, rice vinegar, sugar, peppercorns and chilli powder. Stir-fry for 2 minutes, then add the stock or water and simmer for 2 minutes.

3 Place the steamed rice in the prepared claypot. Spoon the pork and eggplant mixture over the rice and arrange the chopped spinach on top. Cover with the lid.

4 Place the claypot on the cooktop, bring to a high heat for 3 to 4 minutes, then reduce the heat and continue cooking gently for a further 5 minutes or until the edges of the rice are crispy and sizzling. Serve immediately.

Serves per portion
Protein 2   **Carb** 3   **Fat** 1   **Veg** 3

Herbed Fish Parcels with Sweet Potato Wedges and Coleslaw

High in protein and low in fat, this meal is a far cry from fish and chips. It is also loaded with beta-carotene, potassium and magnesium.

Per serve
kJ/Cal 1186/279   **Protein** 34 g   **Fat** 8 g (saturated 1 g)
Carbohydrate 22 g   **Fibre** 5 g   **GI** Low

Preparation time 30 minutes
Cooking time 40 minutes   **Serves** 4

500 g sweet potato, peeled and cut into wedges

spray olive oil

1 teaspoon Cajun spice mix

4 × 150 g white fish fillets

2 teaspoons dill, chopped

2 teaspoons lemon rind, finely grated

freshly ground black pepper, to taste

Coleslaw

250 g cabbage, finely shredded

1 carrot, grated

½ red onion, finely chopped

¼ cup flatleaf parsley, chopped

1 tablespoon whole egg mayonnaise

2 tablespoons lemon juice

1 Preheat the oven to 200°C and line a large baking tray with non-stick baking paper.

2 Spray the sweet potato wedges lightly with oil, and sprinkle with the Cajun spice mix. Toss to coat. Arrange in a single layer on the lined tray, and bake for 25 minutes.

3 Meanwhile, tear 4 squares of non-stick baking paper. Place a fish fillet on each sheet and sprinkle with the dill and lemon rind. Season with pepper. Fold and wrap the baking paper securely to enclose the fish, then place on a baking tray. Add to the oven and cook for 15 minutes (so the sweet potatoes cook for 40 minutes in total).

4 For the coleslaw, combine the cabbage, carrot, onion and parsley in a large bowl. Add the mayonnaise and lemon juice; toss to combine. Serve the coleslaw with the fish and wedges.

Serves per portion
Protein 3   **Carb** 1   **Veg** 1½

Angelhair Pasta with Chilli Seafood Sauce

This recipe will please not only pasta lovers but anyone interested in a nutrient-dense dish, kind to the body and a joy to the palate.

Per serve
kJ/Cal 2170/515 **Protein** 40 g **Fat** 15 g (saturated 2 g)
Carbohydrate 47 g **Fibre** 3 g **GI** Low

Preparation time 15 minutes
Cooking time 35 minutes **Serves** 6

350 g small clams, scrubbed and rinsed

350 g mussels, scrubbed, beards removed, and rinsed

350 g medium-sized prawns, peeled and deveined

350 g scallops

1 tablespoon extra-virgin olive oil

2 large cloves garlic, minced

3 large shallots, finely chopped

3 tablespoons finely chopped flatleaf parsley

¾ cup (200 ml) dry white wine

1 × 400 g can tomatoes

350 g angelhair pasta

chilli flakes, to taste

2 tablespoons extra-virgin olive oil, extra

1 Soak the clams and mussels in cold water for 5 minutes. Discard any with opened shells. Drain and set aside. In a separate bowl, rinse and drain the prawns and scallops. Set aside.

2 In a wide, deep frypan, warm the olive oil, then add the garlic and shallots. Sauté for 1–2 minutes, until the shallots become soft (avoid burning the garlic). Stir in the parsley. Pour in the wine and cook over a medium–high heat for 3 minutes. Add the tomatoes and their liquid. Bring the mixture to a boil, then simmer, uncovered, for 15–20 minutes, stirring frequently.

3 Add the clams and the mussels to the sauce. Once their shells start opening (time varies with size—about 2–6 minutes), add the prawns, scallops and chilli flakes, to taste. Continue cooking for about 3 minutes.

4 Meanwhile, bring about 4 litres of water to the boil. Add the pasta and cook for 2 minutes. Use a wooden spoon to separate the strands. When the pasta is cooked al dente, drain and place in a large, warmed serving bowl. Drizzle the extra olive oil over the pasta and stir thoroughly.

5 Add the sauce to the pasta and mix thoroughly. Serve at once.

Serves per portion
Protein 3   **Carb** 3   **Fat** 1   **Veg** 0.5

Prawn and Mango Salad with Chilli Lime Dressing

This salad is loaded with potassium and is a good source of zinc. The fat it contains is largely monounsaturated. It is best made just before serving.

Per serve
kJ/Cal 1518/357   **Protein** 26 g   **Fat** 13 g (saturated 3 g)
Carbohydrate 31 g   **Fibre** 7 g   **GI** Low

Preparation time 15 minutes
Cooking time 3 minutes (plus cooling time)   **Serves** 4

6 baby potatoes (about 70 g each), quartered

750 g cooked whole prawns, peeled and deveined

100 g snowpea sprouts, ends trimmed

1 cup fresh mint leaves, torn

⅓ cup (80 ml) sweet chilli sauce

¼ cup (60 ml) lime juice

1 mango, flesh cut into short, thin slices

1 avocado, thinly sliced

1 Place the potato in a shallow, microwave-safe dish. Pour over about 2 tablespoons of water, cover, and cook on high for 3 minutes or until tender. Set aside to cool.

2 Place the cooled potatoes, prawns, snowpea sprouts and mint leaves in a bowl and toss to combine.

3 Whisk the sweet chilli sauce and lime juice together for the dressing.

4 Divide the salad among serving plates. Top with the mango and avocado slices. Drizzle over the dressing and serve.

Serves per portion
Protein 2   **Fat** 1   **Carb** 1½   **Veg** 1

Mushroom and Vegetable Stir-fry

Per serve
kJ/Cal 1410/335 **Protein** 9 g **Fat** 3 g (saturated <1 g)
Carbohydrate 65 g **Fibre** 4 g **GI** Moderate

Preparation time 15 minutes
Cooking time 15 minutes **Serves** 4

1½ cups (300 g) Basmati rice, rinsed

1 bunch baby bok choy

2 teaspoons peanut or vegetable oil

1 small red onion, halved and thinly sliced

1 red capsicum, cut into thin strips

250 g mushrooms, sliced

2 garlic cloves, crushed

2 teaspoons ginger, grated

1 teaspoon red chilli, chopped

1 tablespoon salt-reduced soy sauce

1 Bring 2¼ cups of water to the boil in a large, tightly covered saucepan. Stir in the rice and quickly replace the lid. Reduce the heat to as low as possible and cook for 10 minutes. Remove from the heat and leave to stand, still covered, for 5 minutes.

2 Meanwhile, cut the bok choy in half to separate the leaves from the stems. Cut the leaves into wide shreds, and finely slice the stems.

3 Heat the oil in a wok and add the onion. Stir-fry over a moderate-high heat for 2 minutes, until just tender. Add the capsicum and bok choy stems and stir-fry for 3 minutes.

4 Add the mushrooms, garlic, ginger and chilli, and stir-fry for 3 minutes, until the mushrooms are just soft. Drizzle with soy sauce and toss to combine. Serve immediately with the rice.

Serves per portion
Carb 4 **Veg** 3

Moroccan-style Lentil and Vegetable Stew with Couscous

Per serve
kJ/Cal 1172/276   **Protein** 14 g   **Fat** 3 g (saturated <1 g)
Carbohydrate 44 g   **Fibre** 8 g   **GI** Moderate

Preparation time 25 minutes
Cooking time 50 minutes   **Serves** 4

2 teaspoons olive oil	**1** Heat the oil in a large saucepan over a medium heat. Add the onion and cook for 5 minutes until soft and lightly golden. Add the garlic, ginger and spices and cook for 30 seconds, stirring.
1 onion, chopped	
2 cloves garlic, crushed	
2 teaspoons grated fresh ginger	
2 teaspoons ground cumin	**2** Add the stock and tomatoes. Stir to combine, scraping the bottom of the pan. Add the cauliflower, eggplant and beans, stir to combine, and bring to the boil. Reduce the heat to medium–low and simmer, covered, for 30 minutes, until the vegetables are tender. Uncover and cook for a further 10 minutes.
2 teaspoons ground coriander	
1 cup (250 ml) vegetable stock	
1 × 400 g can chopped tomatoes	
400 g cauliflower, cut into small florets	
1 eggplant, cut into 2 cm cubes	**3** Stir in the lentils and cook for 5 minutes to heat through.
150 g green beans, cut into 4 cm lengths	**4** Meanwhile, bring 1¼ cups (310 ml) of water to the boil in a medium-size saucepan. Add the couscous, cover tightly and turn off the heat. Leave to stand for 5 minutes, then uncover and fluff up the grains with a fork.
1 × 400 g can green lentils, rinsed and drained	
1 cup (150 g) couscous	
	5 Serve the spicy vegetable stew over the couscous.

Serves per portion
Protein ½   **Carb** 1   **Veg** 3½

Tagine of Sweet Potato, Pumpkin, Prunes and Chickpeas

This is a delicious vegetarian dish that can be put together when there isn't much in the fridge. Serve it on its own or with couscous or rice if you wish.

Per serve
kJ/Cal 1210/290   **Protein** 11 g   **Fat** 7 g (saturated 1 g)
Carbohydrate 42 g   **Fibre** 10 g   **GI** Medium

Preparation time 15 minutes
Cooking time 30 minutes   **Serves** 4

1 tablespoon olive oil
1 onion, finely chopped
1 garlic clove, crushed
1 teaspoon ground cumin
1 teaspoon ground coriander
½ teaspoon turmeric
300 g sweet potato, peeled and cut into 2 cm chunks
300 g butternut pumpkin, peeled and cut into 2 cm chunks
1 × 400 g can diced tomatoes in tomato juice
1 cup (250 ml) vegetable stock
1 × 400 g can chickpeas, drained
100 g pitted prunes
2 medium-sized zucchinis, sliced into rounds

1 Heat the oil in a large frypan over a medium heat, add the onion and garlic and sauté lightly for about 3 minutes or until soft and golden. Add the cumin, coriander and turmeric and stir until aromatic.

2 Add the sweet potato and pumpkin and stir to coat in the spices. Stir in the tomatoes, stock and chickpeas. Cover and simmer gently for 15 minutes, then add the prunes and zucchini. Cover and simmer for a further 10 minutes, or until all the vegetables are tender.

3 Serve with couscous or Basmati rice.

Serves per portion
Carb 2   **Veg** 3   **Fruit** 1

Chickpea Curry

Per serve
kJ/Cal 910/215   **Protein** 10 g   **Fat** 8 g (saturated <1 g)
Carbohydrate 23 g   **Fibre** 8 g   **GI** Low

Preparation time 10 minutes
Cooking time about 30 minutes   **Serves** 4–6

1 tablespoon canola oil
1 large onion, finely chopped
1 clove garlic, finely diced
1 teaspoon finely grated ginger
2 tomatoes, chopped
1 teaspoon ground cumin
1 teaspoon ground cloves, or to taste
3 teaspoons ground coriander
3 teaspoons ground chilli, or to taste
salt to taste (optional)
2 × 400 g cans chickpeas, drained
¾ cup water
2 teaspoons tamarind paste
freshly ground black pepper, to taste
2 teaspoons garam masala
1 teaspoon sugar

1 Heat the oil in a heavy-based pan and gently cook the onions until soft and golden (about 5 minutes). Add the garlic and ginger and cook for a further 5 minutes, then add the chopped tomatoes, cumin, cloves, coriander and chilli. Season with salt if desired.

2 Add the chickpeas and water and bring to the boil, then reduce the heat and stir in the tamarind paste, pepper, garam masala and sugar. Simmer uncovered for 15 minutes. Serve hot.

Serves per portion
Carb 1   **Veg** 1

Savoury snacks and sweet treats

Herbed Salmon Spread

This spread is rich in omega-3 fats and delicious with grainy crackers or low-GI bread. If you prefer, you could replace the salmon with tuna. It will keep in the refrigerator for up to three days.

Per serve
kJ/Cal 637/150   **Protein** 15 g   **Fat** 10 g (saturated 4 g)
Carbohydrate 1 g   **Fibre** <1 g   **GI** Low

Preparation time 10 minutes
Cooking time nil   **Serves** 4

1 × 200 g can salmon (red or pink) in spring water, drained

1 × 200 g reduced-fat fresh ricotta

½ teaspoon lemon rind, finely grated

2 teaspoons lemon juice

1 tablespoon chives, chopped

1 tablespoon flatleaf parsley, chopped

salt and freshly ground black pepper, to taste

1 Place the salmon in a bowl and flake with a fork. Add the ricotta, lemon rind and juice and herbs. Mash with a fork until well combined.

2 Season to taste.

Serves per portion
Protein 1   **Fat** 1

Bruschetta with Basil and Tomatoes

Per serve

kJ/Cal 429/101   **Protein** 4 g   **Fat** 1 g (saturated <1 g)
Carbohydrate 18 g   **Fibre** 3 g   **GI** Low

Preparation time 10 minutes
Cooking time about 5 minutes   **Makes** 4

4 slices sourdough bread (preferably day-old)

1 garlic clove, peeled and halved

2 medium tomatoes, diced

½ small red onion, finely chopped

¼ cup basil leaves, shredded

1 teaspoon balsamic vinegar (optional)

salt and freshly ground pepper, to taste

1 Toast the bread on both sides until golden brown. Rub with the cut garlic clove, and set aside to cool.

2 Combine the tomatoes with the onion and basil. Drizzle with the balsamic vinegar (optional) and season with salt and pepper.

3 Spoon the tomato mixture onto the sourdough toast slices and serve immediately.

Serves per portion
Carb 1   **Veg** ½

Eggplant and Bean Purée

This eggplant purée is a nutritious and tasty addition to sandwiches, or can be enjoyed spread on grainy crackers or wholemeal pita bread.

Per serve
kJ/Cal 320/75   **Protein** 5 g
Fat 3 g (saturated <1 g)   **Carbohydrate** 6 g
Fibre 5 g   **GI** Low

Per serve (with vegetables)
kJ/Cal 320/75   **Protein** 5 g
Fat 3 g (saturated <1 g)   **Carbohydrate** 6 g
Fibre 5 g   **GI** Low

Preparation time 20 minutes
Cooking time 40 minutes (plus cooling time)   **Serves** 6

1 large eggplant (about 400 g), cut in half lengthways

1 × 400 g can soybeans, rinsed and drained

1 teaspoon ground cumin

1 clove garlic, crushed

2 tablespoons lemon juice

1 red capsicum, cut into sticks

1 Lebanese cucumber, cut into rounds

1 carrot, cut into sticks

1 Preheat the oven to 190°C and line a baking tray with lightly oiled foil.

2 Place the eggplant cut side down on the foil. Bake for 35 minutes, until the eggplant is soft.

3 Cool the eggplant until just warm, then scoop the flesh out of the skin and place in a food processor. Add the soybeans, cumin, garlic and lemon juice, and process until smooth.

4 Serve with the vegetables for dipping.

Serves per portion
Carb ½   **Veg** ½ (1½ with vegetables)

Apricot and Almond Cookies

These cookies will keep in an airtight container for three to four days.

Per two cookies
kJ/Cal 760/180   **Protein** 4 g   **Fat** 8 g (saturated <2 g)
Carbohydrate 26 g   **Fibre** 2 g   **GI** Low

Preparation time 15 minutes
Cooking time 15 minutes   **Makes** about 16 cookies

100 g dried apricots, diced
100 g almond meal
½ cup (115 g) caster sugar
⅓ cup (50 g) plain flour
2 egg whites, at room
temperature

1 Preheat the oven to 170°C and line two baking trays with non-stick baking paper.

2 Place the apricots, almond meal, sugar and flour in a bowl and mix well to combine.

3 Whisk the egg whites until frothy. Add to the apricot mixture and mix until well combined.

4 Use slightly wet hands to shape tablespoonfuls of the mixture into balls. Place on the lined trays and use a spoon to press out slightly.

5 Bake for 12–15 minutes, swapping the trays around once, until the biscuits are set and light golden on the bottom. Leave to cool on the trays for 5 minutes before transferring to a wire rack to cool completely.

Serves per portion
Carb 1   **Fat** 1   **Fruit** 1

Muesli and Honey Slice

This slice will keep in an airtight container for three to four days.

Per piece
kJ/Cal 650/153   **Protein** 3 g   **Fat** 7g (saturated 1 g)
Carbohydrate 21 g   **Fibre** 2 g   **GI** Low

Preparation time 10 minutes
Cooking time 20–25 minutes   **Makes** 16 pieces

½ cup (125 ml) honey
100 g monounsaturated, salt-reduced margarine
2 eggs
2 cups (240 g) natural muesli
½ cup (75 g) self-raising flour

1 Preheat the oven to 170°C and line a 16 × 26 cm slab pan with non-stick baking paper.

2 Place the honey and margarine in a small saucepan. Stir over a low heat until the margarine melts and the mixture is well combined. Set aside to cool. Pour into a bowl and whisk in the eggs.

3 Combine the muesli and flour in a bowl. Add the cooled honey mixture and stir well to combine. Pour into the lined pan and smooth the surface. Bake for 20–25 minutes or until set and golden. Set aside in the pan to cool.

4 Cut the slice into 16 pieces. Store in an airtight container.

Serves per portion
Carb 1   **Fat** ½

Banana and Ricotta Toasts

Other fruity toppings for ricotta toasts include sliced strawberries, peach or nectarine slices and pear slices with walnuts.

Per serve
kJ/Cal 727/171   **Protein** 6 g   **Fat** 3 g (saturated 2 g)
Carbohydrate 29 g   **Fibre** 3 g   **GI** Low

Preparation time 5 minutes
Cooking time 5 minutes   **Makes** 4 toasts

100 g low-fat fresh ricotta
1 tablespoon honey
pinch ground cinnamon
4 slices grainy bread
2 small bananas, diagonally sliced
extra honey, to serve
extra cinnamon, to serve

1 Use electric beaters to beat the ricotta, honey and cinnamon until almost smooth.

2 Toast the bread until golden.

3 Spread the ricotta mixture evenly on the bread.

4 Top with the bananas. Drizzle over a little extra honey and a sprinkle of cinnamon and serve immediately.

Serves per portion
Protein ½   **Carb** 1   **Fruit** ½

Fruit Parfaits

If you like, use low-fat vanilla yoghurt instead of Frûche. The almond bread referred to is a very thin, sweet biscuit, similar to Italian biscotti, but wafer-thin. It is available from the biscuit or gourmet section of the supermarket.

Per serve
kJ/Cal 1090/256   **Protein** 12 g   **Fat** 4 g (saturated <1 g)
Carbohydrate 38 g   **Fibre** 4 g   **GI** Low

Preparation time 20 minutes
Refrigeration time 30 minutes   **Makes** 4 parfaits

150 g raspberries (fresh or thawed frozen)

1 tablespoon orange juice

90 g almond bread

4 nectarines or peaches, sliced

400 g vanilla reduced-fat fromage frais (Frûche)

1 Place the raspberries in a bowl, then add the orange juice. Mash with a fork, and stir to make a chunky sauce.

2 Break the almond bread into bite-size pieces. Layer the nectarines (or peaches), raspberry sauce, almond bread and fromage frais in parfait glasses.

3 To let the flavours blend, refrigerate the parfaits for 30 minutes before serving.

Serves per portion
Protein 1   **Carb** ½   **Fruit** 1

Blueberry Cheesecakes

Per serve

kJ/Cal 875/206   **Protein** 10 g   **Fat** 13 g (saturated 5 g)
Carbohydrate 12 g   **Fibre** 2 g   **GI** Low

Preparation time 20 minutes
Refrigeration time 1 hour   **Makes** 4 cheesecakes

300 g low-fat ricotta
1 tablespoon honey
1 teaspoon finely grated orange rind
1 cup (150 g) fresh blueberries
⅓ cup (40 g) walnuts, finely chopped
4 strawberries, sliced

1 Line 4 × ½ cup (125 ml) capacity ramekins with plastic wrap.

2 Place the ricotta, honey and orange rind in a bowl and mash with a fork.

3 Combine two-thirds of the blueberries with the ricotta mixture and divide between the ramekins. Press in firmly and smooth the surface.

4 Sprinkle over the walnuts. Smooth out with the back of a spoon and press the nuts into the mixture. Refrigerate for 1 hour, to firm and chill.

5 To serve, invert onto a plate and peel away the plastic wrap. Top each cake with a sliced strawberry, and serve with the remaining blueberries.

Serves per portion
Protein 1   **Fat** 1   **Fruit** ½

Creamed Rice with Rhubarb and Strawberries

There is almost no fat in this dessert. The rhubarb mixture will keep in an airtight container in the refrigerator for three to four days.

Per serve
kJ/Cal 1030/242   **Protein** 8 g   **Fat** 0 g
Carbohydrate 50 g   **Fibre** 4 g   **GI** Low

Preparation time 10 minutes (plus cooling time)
Cooking time 25 minutes   **Serves** 4

1 bunch rhubarb, ends trimmed and cut into 3 cm pieces
¼ cup (55 g) caster sugar
1 punnet strawberries, hulled and halved
½ cup (100 g) Doongara CleverRice
2 tablespoons caster sugar, extra
2 cups (500 ml) skim milk
pinch ground cinnamon

1   Place the rhubarb and sugar in a medium-size, heavy-based saucepan. Stir constantly over a medium heat for 5 minutes until the rhubarb starts to soften. Add the strawberries and cook for a further 5 minutes or until the rhubarb and strawberries are tender. Remove from the heat and set aside to cool.

2   Meanwhile, place the rice, extra sugar and 1¼ cups (310 ml) of the skim milk in another medium-size, heavy-based saucepan. Stir over a low heat until the sugar dissolves, then increase the heat and bring to a simmer. Reduce the heat to low, cover, and cook for 12 minutes.

3   Remove from the heat and stir in the remaining milk, then cover and set aside for 10 minutes. Stir in a pinch of cinnamon and serve with the rhubarb mixture.

Serves per protein
Protein ½   **Carb** 1   **Fruit** 1

Orange and Passionfruit Mousse

This dessert is a good source of calcium and phosphorus and contains less than 1 gram of fat per serve. It will keep in the refrigerator for up to two days.

Per serve
kJ/Cal 505/119   **Protein** 7 g   **Fat** <1 g (saturated <1 g)
Carbohydrate 23 g   **Fibre** 1 g   **GI** Low

Preparation time 15 minutes
Cooking time 2 minutes (plus chilling and setting time)   **Serves** 6

⅔ cup (160 ml) freshly squeezed orange juice

⅓ cup (80 g) caster sugar

2 teaspoons powdered gelatine

⅓ cup (80 ml) fresh passionfruit pulp

1 × 375 ml can light evaporated milk, chilled

extra passionfruit, to serve (optional)

1 Place the orange juice and sugar in a small saucepan. Heat until hot, not boiling. Remove from the heat and stir in the gelatine until it dissolves. Pour the mixture into a small heatproof bowl and set aside to cool slightly. Stir in the passionfruit pulp.

2 In a large bowl use electric beaters to whisk the evaporated milk until light and fluffy. Add the orange juice mixture and stir to combine. Cover the bowl and chill for 1–1½ hours, stirring often, or until the mousse starts to thicken and set slightly. (Stirring will help the passionfruit to suspend in the mousse rather than sinking to the bottom.)

3 Spoon the mousse mixture into individual serving dishes. Refrigerate for a further 3–4 hours or until set.

4 Serve the mousse drizzled with extra passionfruit, if desired.

Serves per protein
Protein ½   **Fruit** ½

The GI Tables

THE FOLLOWING TABLES GIVE A COMPREHENSIVE UP-TO-date listing of the GI of hundreds of popular foods in alphabetical order. These tables will help you put those low-GI food choices into your shopping trolley and onto your plate. Each entry lists an individual food and its GI value. We also list the nominal serving size, the amount of carbohydrate per serving, the GL, and whether the food's GI is low, medium or high.

High, Medium, or Low GI . . .

- A high GI value is 70 or more.
- A medium/moderate GI value is 56-69 inclusive.
- A low GI value is 55 or less.

You can use the tables to:
- find the GI of your favourite foods
- compare carb-rich foods within a category (two types of bread or breakfast cereal, for example)

- identify the best carbohydrate choices
- improve your diet by finding a low–GI substitute for high-GI foods
- put together a low–GI meal
- find foods with a high GI but low GL.

Each individual food appears alphabetically within a food category, such as 'Bread' or 'Fruit'. This makes it easy to compare the kinds of foods you eat every day and helps you see which high-GI foods you can replace with low-GI versions.

In the tables you will sometimes see these symbols:

★ indicates that a food contains very little or no carbohydrate which means that the GI isn't relevant (or can't be tested). You will find this symbol beside foods like cheese, fish, chicken, meat and green leafy vegetables. We have included these foods because so many people ask us for their GI.

■ indicates that a food is high in saturated fat.

● indicates that a food does contain carbohydrate but has either not been GI tested or the results of the testing have not been published. To help you manage your blood glucose levels and reduce the overall GI of your diet you will find this symbol in these tables besides products like biscuits and cereals – carb-rich foods that we regularly buy. Although it's not possible to work out an accurate GI value for a product based on its ingredients, it is possible to make an educated guess as to whether it will be high or low GI, based on similar products that have been tested.

ⓖ indicates that a food is part of the GI Symbol Program. Foods with the GI symbol have had their GI tested properly and are a healthy choice for their food category.

To make a fair comparison, all foods have been tested using an internationally standardised method. Gram for gram of carbohydrates, the higher the GI, the higher the blood glucose levels after consumption. If you can't find the GI value in these tables for a food you eat regularly, check out our web site (www.glycemicindex.com), where we maintain an international database of published GI values that have been tested by a reliable laboratory. Alternatively, please write to the manufacturer and encourage them to have the food tested by an accredited laboratory. In the meantime, choose a similar food from the tables as a substitute.

The GI values in this book are correct at the time of publication. However, the formulation of commercial foods can change and the GI may change as well. You can rely on foods showing the GI symbol. Although some manufacturers include the GI on the nutritional label, you would need to know that the testing was carried out independently by an accredited laboratory.

GISP	FOOD	GI	SAMPLE SERVING	AVAILABLE CARB (G) PER SERVE	GL PER SERVE
	SWEET BISCUITS — LOW GI (LESS THAN OR EQUAL TO 55)				
	Arnott's				
	Snack Right varieties (apple & sultana, wild berry, fruit pillow)	45–52	2 biscuits, 33g	24	12
	Snack Right sultana, fruit slice	48–52	2 biscuits, 20g	22	11
	Snack Right sultana, choc fruit slice	45	2 biscuits, 25g	17	8
	Carman's Apricot and Almond Rounds	46	1 serve, 40g	22	10
	Carman's Classic Fruit & Nut Rounds	42	1 serve, 40g	23	9
	Maltmeal Wafer, Griffins NZ	50	2 biscuits, 25g	17	9
	Generic				
	Chocolate chip cookies (made with coconut flour)	43 ■	2 biscuits, 20g	16	7
	Coconut macaroons	32	2 biscuits, 20g	1	4
	100 Healthy Calories Fruit Cookies, Freedom Foods	47	2 biscuits, 25g	19	9
	Maltmeal Wafer, Griffins NZ	50	2 biscuits, 25g	17	9
	Oatmeal, Highland	55	2 biscuits, 20g	14	8
	Oatmeal	54	2 biscuits, 20g	14	8
	Rich tea	55	2 biscuits, 20g	13	7
	SWEET BISCUITS — HIGHER GI (MORE THAN 55 OR UNKNOWN) **(LESS THAN 10% TOTAL FAT, LESS THAN 1.5g SAT FAT/SERVE)**				
	Arnott's				
	Choc Ripple	•	2 biscuits, 18g	13	•
	Chocolate Royals, dark chocolate	•	1 biscuit, 17g	11	•
	Chocolate Royals, milk chocolate	•	1 biscuit, 17g	11	•
	Chocolate, Teddy Bear	•	1 biscuit, 17g	11	•
	Chocolate, Tee Vee Snacks	•	4 biscuits, 20g	13	•
	Full o' Fruit	•	2 biscuits, 20g	15	•
	Ginger Nut	•	1 biscuit, 13g	11	•
	Golden Fruit, Griffins NZ	77	2 biscuits, 25g	17	13
	Honey Jumbles	•	2 biscuits, 20g	16	•

★ little or no carbs ■ high in saturated fat ● untested/unknown Ⓖ GI Symbol partner

GISP	FOOD	GI	SAMPLE SERVING	AVAILABLE CARB (G) PER SERVE	GL PER SERVE
	Hundreds & Thousands	•	2 biscuits, 17g	13	•
	Malt-O-Milk	•	3 biscuits, 21g	16	•
	Marie	•	2 biscuits, 16g	12	•
	Milk Arrowroot	69	2 biscuits, 16g	12	8
	Milk Coffee	•	2 biscuits, 17g	13	•
	Morning Coffee	79	3 biscuits, 17g	12	9
	Scalliwag	•	2 biscuits, 20g	15	•
	Shredded Wheatmeal	62	3 biscuits, 23g	15	9
	Spicy Fruit Roll	•	1 biscuit, 17g	12	•
	Teddy Bear	•	2 biscuits, 21g	15	•
	Tic Toc	•	2 biscuits, 18g	13	•
	Paradise				
	Vive Lites, caramel pecan	•	2 biscuits, 21g	16	•
	Vive Lites, choc chip mini cookies	•	1 mini pack, 30g	24	•
	Vive Wellbeing, date & ginger	•	2 biscuits, 18g	13	•
	Weight Watchers				
	Butternut	•	2 biscuits, 18g	14	•
	Fruit Slice	•	2 cookies, 23g	17	•
	Triple Choc	•	2 biscuits, 18g	11	•
	Generic				
	Shortbread, plain	64 ■	2 biscuits, 25g	16	10
	Vanilla wafer, cream-filled	77 ■	3 biscuits, 25g	18	14
SAVOURY BISCUITS – LOW GI (LESS THAN OR EQUAL TO 55)					
	Arnott's				
	Jatz	55	6 crackers, 25g	13	7
	Shapes, barbecue	48	10 crackers, 23g	15	7
	Vita-Wheat Lunch Slices Soy, Linseed & Sesame	52	2 slices, 38g	22	11
	Ryvita varieties				
Ⓖ	Pumpkin Seeds & Oats crispbread	46	2 slices, 25g	14	6
Ⓖ	Sunflower Seeds & Oats crispbread	48	2 slices, 25g	14	7

★ little or no carbs   ■ high in saturated fat   ● untested/unknown   Ⓖ GI Symbol partner

GISP	FOOD	GI	SAMPLE SERVING	AVAILABLE CARB (G) PER SERVE	GL PER SERVE
	SAVOURY BISCUITS – HIGHER GI (MORE THAN 55 OR UNKNOWN)				
	Arnott's				
	Breton	67 ■	6 crackers, 26g	15	10
	Cruskits varieties				
	Corn	•	4 crackers, 19g	14	•
	Light	•	4 crackers, 23g	17	•
	Rye	•	4 crackers, 19g	12	•
	Jatz 97% fat free	•	5 crackers, 19g	15	•
	Salada varieties				
	Light original	•	1 cracker, 14g	11	•
	Light poppy & sesame	•	1 cracker, 14g	11	•
	Multigrain 97% fat free	•	1 cracker, 14g	11	•
	Original	•	1 cracker, 14g	10	•
	Wholemeal	•	1 cracker, 14g	9	•
	Generic				
	Sao	70 ■	3 crackers, 26g	16	11
	Thin Captain	•	3 crackers, 17g	12	•
	Vita-Weat varieties				
	9-Grain	•	2 sandwich, 23g	15	•
	9-Grain	•	4 regular, 25g	14	•
	Cracked Pepper	•	4 regular, 23g	16	•
	Grain Snacks, all varieties	•	1 packet, 20g	13	•
	Grain Sticks	•	1 packet, 20g	13	•
	Lunch Slices, Sunflower, Pumpkin & Canola	59	2 slices, 38g	22	13
	Original	•	4 regular, 25g	16	•
	Sesame	•	4 regular, 23g	13	•
	Soy & Linseed	•	4 regular, 23g	13	•
	Water cracker	78	6 crackers, 18g	14	11

★ little or no carbs　■ high in saturated fat　● untested/unknown　Ⓖ GI Symbol partner

GISP	FOOD	GI	SAMPLE SERVING	AVAILABLE CARB (G) PER SERVE	GL PER SERVE
	Paradise				
	Vive Lites Wholemeal crispbread	•	4 biscuits, 28g	20	•
	Vive Wellbeing 7 Grains crispbread	•	4 biscuits, 32g	20	•
	Generic				
	Rice cake, puffed	82	2 slices, 20g	15	12
	Rice cracker	91	12 crackers, 20g	16	15

GISP	FOOD	GI	SAMPLE SERVING	AVAILABLE CARB (G) PER SERVE	GL PER SERVE
	BREAD & BAKERY PRODUCTS – LOW GI (LESS THAN OR EQUAL TO 55)				
	Bakers Delight				
	Cape Seed				
	Loaf	48	1 toast slice, 45g	13	6
	Roll	48	89g	27	13
	Cape Fruit & Nut roll	55	89g	33	18
	Wholemeal Country Grain				
	Block loaf	53	1 toast slice, 40g	15	8
	Dinner roll	53	34g	13	7
	Long roll	53	65g	27	14
	Round roll	53	65g	27	14
	Bill's Bakery				
	Sourdough Multigrain	•	1 slice, 35g	15	•
	Bürgen				
©	Fruit & Muesli	53	1 slice, 42g	19	10
©	Pumpkin Seeds	51	1 slice, 42g	11	6
©	Rye	53	1 slice, 42g	14	7
©	Soy-Lin	52	1 slice, 42g	13	7
©	Wholemeal with Seeds	39	1 slice, 42g	9	4
	Buttercup				
	Fruit & Spice loaf	54	1 thick slice, 30g	15	8
	Country Life varieties				
	Low GI Gluten free, white	53	1 slice, 32g	19	10
	Diego's				
	White corn tortillas	53	1 regular, 56g	27	14
	Reduced carb wraps	51	1 regular, 43g	11	6
	Golden Hearth				
	Heavy Wholegrain Organic	53	1 large slice, 50g	21	11
	Pav's Bakery				
	Spelt Multigrain	54	1 slice, 30g	12	7

★ little or no carbs ■ high in saturated fat ● untested/unknown © GI Symbol partner

GISP	FOOD	GI	SAMPLE SERVING	AVAILABLE CARB (G) PER SERVE	GL PER SERVE
	Tip-Top varieties				
Ⓖ	9-Grain Original	53	1 slice, 37g	13	7
Ⓖ	9-Grain Pumpkin Seed	52	1 slice, 37g	13	7
Ⓖ	9-Grain Wholemeal	53	1 slice, 38g	12	6
	Spicy Fruit loaf	54	1 slice, 36g	19	10
	Woolworth's Select				
	Traditional white corn tortilla	53	1 regular, 56g	27	14
	Reduced carb tortilla	51	1 regular, 43g	16	8
	Specialty breads				
	Continental fruit	47	1 thick slice, 45g	24	11
	Pumpernickel	50	1 slice, 47g	21	11
	Sourdough, wheat	54	1 large slice, 64g	33	18
	Sourdough, rye	48	1 large slice, 64g	28	13

BREAD & BAKERY PRODUCTS –
HIGHER GI (MORE THAN 55 OR UNKNOWN)

GISP	FOOD	GI	SAMPLE SERVING	AVAILABLE CARB (G) PER SERVE	GL PER SERVE
	Bakers Delight				
	Apricot Delight				
	Log	56	1 slice, 43g	24	13
	Roll	56	80g	48	27
	Scroll	56	105g	60	34
	Authentic sourdough				
	Loaf	58	1 toast slice, 33g	16	9
	Roll	58	115g	59	34
	Block loaf, wholemeal	71	1 toast slice, 38g	14	10
	Chia, white	63	1 toast slice, 40g	17	11
	Country Grain loaf	61	1 toast slice, 38g	19	12
	Soy & Linseed loaf	59	1 toast slice, 48g	14	8
	Tiger loaf, white	71	1 toast slice, 37g	17	12
	Toasty Fruit loaf	61	1 toast slice, 37g	25	15
	Country Life				
	Gluten free, multigrain	79	1 slice, 30g	13	10

★ little or no carbs ■ high in saturated fat ● untested/unknown Ⓖ GI Symbol partner

GISP	FOOD	GI	SAMPLE SERVING	AVAILABLE CARB (G) PER SERVE	GL PER SERVE
	Naturis				
	Gluten free, buckwheat	72	1 slice, 48g	17	12
	Noble Rise				
	Sourdough White	79	1 slice, 30g	12	9
	Tip-Top				
	EnerGI, white sandwich	58	1 slice, 37g	17	10
	Raisin toast, Retreats	63	1 slice, 33g	19	12
	Sunblest, white	71	1 slice, 30g	14	10
	Sunblest, wholemeal	71	1 slice, 30g	12	9
	Wonder White				
	Wonder White Lower GI	59	1 slice, 35g	13	8
	Specialty Breads & Baked Foods				
	Bagel	72	1 large, 85g	43	31
	Baguette, traditional French	77	¼ loaf, 62g	33	25
	Breadcrumbs, white		¼ loaf, 30g	20	●
	Chapatti, corn	59	1 small, 35g	14	8
	Chapatti, bajra	49	1 regular, 100g	14	7
	Chapatti, barley	48	1 regular, 100g	14	8
	Croissant	67	1 large, 70g	24	16
	Crumpet, white	69	100g	42	29
	Golden mini-finger crumpets	69	30g	13	9
	Golden round crumpets	69	50g	16	11
	Golden square crumpet breaks	69	70g	23	16
	Doughnut, commercial, cinnamon	75	1 regular, 50g	25	30
	English muffin	77	1 regular, 64g	23	18
	Foccacia	●	1 piece, 50g	21	●
	Fruit	●	1 slice, 31g	16	●
	Fruit bun, iced	●	1 regular, 85g	39	●
	Gluten free, commercial	●	1 medium slice, 30g	16	●
	Hamburger bun	61	1 regular, 90g	45	27
	Hotdog bun, white	68	1 regular, 62g	33	22

★ little or no carbs ■ high in saturated fat ● untested/unknown Ⓖ GI Symbol partner

GISP	FOOD	GI	SAMPLE SERVING	AVAILABLE CARB (G) PER SERVE	GL PER SERVE
	Hot cross bun, fruit	•	1 regular, 85g	49	•
	Hot cross bun, choc chip	•	1 regular, 65g	41	•
	Italian bread	73	1 slice, 40g	18	13
	Italian breadsticks, grissini	•	3 sticks, 25g	18	•
	Lavash, white	•	1 piece, 67g	36	•
	Lavash, wholemeal	•	1 piece, 67g	33	•
	Kaiser roll, white	73	1 regular, 108g	60	44
	Lebanese bread, wholemeal	•	1 large, 100g	48	•
	Lebanese bread, white, Seda Bakery	75	1 large, 100g	53	40
	Matzo, Jewish bread	•	1 piece, 30g	24	•
	Melba toast, plain	70	30g	23	16
	Middle Eastern flatbread	91	30g	17	16
	Multigrain	65	1 slice, 34g	15	10
	Naan	•	1 piece, 15cm diam.	46	•
	Wrap, Mountain	•	1 piece 25g	14	•
	Pancakes, buckwheat, gluten free, packet mix, Orgran	102	1/10 pkt, 37.5g	29	30
	Pancakes, gluten-free, packet mix, Freedom Foods	61	1 serve, 80g	53	32
	Pancakes, homemade	•	1 regular, 56g	16	•
	Pancakes, shaker mix, Green's	67	1 regular, 50g	23	15
	Pappadum, microwaved	•	4 regular, 24g	11	•
	Pikelets, homemade	•	4 regular, 100g	48	•
	Pikelets, commercial, Golden	85	1 regular, 25g	9	8
	Pikelets, shake mix	•	1 regular, 35g	16	•
	Pita bread, white	57	1 regular, 60g	33	19
	Roll, white	71	1 regular, 65g	34	24
	Roll, white, dinner	71	1 small, 30g	16	11
	Roll, wholemeal	70	1 regular, 65g	26	18
	Roll, cheese & bacon	•	1 regular, 75g	27	•

★ little or no carbs ■ high in saturated fat ● untested/unknown © GI Symbol partner

GISP	FOOD	GI	SAMPLE SERVING	AVAILABLE CARB (G) PER SERVE	GL PER SERVE
	Rye bread, light	68	1 slice, 30g	14	10
	Rye bread, dark	76	1 slice, 30g	13	10
	Rye bread, wholemeal	58	1 slice, 30g	13	8
	Scone, plain, homemade	•	1 regular, 40g	16	•
	Scone, plain, packet mix, Defiance	92	1 regular, 40g	16	15
	Scone, fruit	•	1 regular, 40g	22	•
	Sliced bread, white	71	1 slice, 32g	14	10
	Sliced bread, wholemeal	71	1 slice, 32g	12	9
	Stuffing, bread	74	100g	22	16
	Taco shell, corn	68	1 large, 20g	11	7
	Turkish pide	87	1 small roll, 85g	40	35
	Waffles, plain	76	1 regular, 33g	19	14

★ little or no carbs ■ high in saturated fat ● untested/unknown Ⓖ GI Symbol partner

GISP	FOOD	GI	SAMPLE SERVING	AVAILABLE CARB (G) PER SERVE	GL PER SERVE
	BREAKFAST CEREALS –				
	LOW GI (LESS THAN OR EQUAL TO 55)				
	Be Natural				
	Cashew, Almond, Hazelnut & Coconut Muesli	54	45g	27	15
	Multi-Grain Porridge	53	40g	22	12
	Pink Lady Apple & Flame Raisin Muesli	51	45g	31	16
	Carman's Classic				
	Fruit Muesli	42	45g	24	10
	Deluxe Fruit Muesli	51	35g	19	10
	Natural Bircher Muesli	40	45g	20	8
	Original Recipe Fruit-Free Muesli	42	45g	23	10
	Generic				
	Oat Bran, raw, unprocessed	55	⅓ cup, 30g	15	8
	Natural muesli	40	½ cup, 45g	27	11
	Porridge, steel-cut oats with water	52	¾ cup, 170g	17	9
	Rice Bran, extruded	19	⅓ cup, 30g	14	3
	Semolina, cooked	55	1 cup, 245g	17	9
	Kellogg's				
	All-Bran	44	¾ cup, 45g	20	9
	Frosties	55	¾ cup, 30g	27	15
	Guardian	37	⅔ cup, 30g	19	7
	Special K Original	53	¾ cup, 30g	21	11
	Sustain	55	¾ cup, 45g	33	18
	Freedom Foods				
	Gluten-free muesli	39	40g	13	5
	Hi-Lite	54	100g	68	37
	Yeast-free muesli	44	40g	13	6
	Goodness Superfoods				
	Digestive 1st	39	45g	21	8
	FibreBoost Sprinkles	34	30g	19	6

★ little or no carbs ■ high in saturated fat ● untested/unknown Ⓖ GI Symbol partner

GISP	FOOD	GI	SAMPLE SERVING	AVAILABLE CARB (G) PER SERVE	GL PER SERVE
	Heart 1st	46	45g	20	9
	Protein 1st	36	45g	17	6
	Quick Sachets Barley + Oats 1st: Apple & Honey Porridge	55	35g serve prepared with water	25	14
	Traditional Barley + Oats 1st: Porridge	47	40g serve prepared with water	25	12
	Monster Muesli				
	Multi-Grain porridge	55	60g	35	19
	Morning Sun				
☉	Apricot & Almond muesli	49	⅔ cup, 60g	34	17
☉	Fruit-free muesli, nuts & seeds	55	⅔ cup, 60g	30	17
☉	Peach & Pecan muesli	49	⅔ cup, 60g	38	19
	Sanitarium				
	Natural muesli	49	30g	19	10
	Vogel's				
	Grain Clusters, classic	54	45g	29	15
	Muesli Cluster Spice	51	45g	27	14
	Muesli Fruit & Nut	48	45g	24	12
	Ultra-Bran	45	45g	22	10
	Woolworth's Select				
	Natural Swiss Bircher muesli	52	½ cup, 50g	30	16
	Naytura Fruit & Nut muesli	48	30g	14	7
	**BREAKFAST CEREALS – HIGHER GI (MORE THAN 55 OR UNKNOWN)**				
	Carman's				
	Traditional Australian Oats, made with water	60	45g serve prepared with water	28	17
	Freedom Foods				
	Quick Oats porridge	●	100g	62	●
	Generic				
	Buckwheat, puffed	65	14g	12	8
	Porridge, regular, oats with water	58	1 cup, 260g	21	12
	Rice porridge	88	100g	9	8

★ little or no carbs ■ high in saturated fat ● untested/unknown ☉ GI Symbol partner

GISP	FOOD	GI	SAMPLE SERVING	AVAILABLE CARB (G) PER SERVE	GL PER SERVE
	Shredded wheat	75	1 biscuit, 24g	16	12
	Traditional rolled oats	57	30g	18	10
	Wheat flake	69	1 biscuit, 15g	10	7
Lowan					
	Fusion muesli, all varieties	•	45g	26–28	•
	Grizzlies	•	35g	26	•
	Honey O's	•	35g	29	•
	Muesli, all varieties	•	45g	26–28	•
	Quick Oats	•	30g	18	•
	Rice Flakes	•	55g	41	•
	Rice Porridge	•	50g	34	•
	Rolled Oats	59	½ cup, 50g	31	18
Kellogg's					
All-Bran varieties					
	Wheat Flakes	•	⅔ cup, 30g	21	13
	Wheat Flakes, honey almond	•	½ cup, 40g	24	•
	Corn Flakes	77	30g	25	19
	Crispix	87	1 cup, 30g	26	23
Crunchy Nut varieties					
	Corn Flakes	72	⅔ cup, 30g	25	18
	Clusters	•	⅔ cup, 30g	23	•
	Froot Loops	69	¾ cup, 30g	26	18
Just Right					
	Original	60	¾ cup, 45g	32	19
Mini-Wheats varieties					
	Blackcurrant	72	⅔ cup, 40g	28	20
	5 Grains, no fruit filling	58	¾ cup, 40g	27	16
	Nutri-Grain	66	1 cup, 30g	21	14
	Rice Bubbles	87	1 cup, 30g	26	23
Special K varieties					
	Advantage	•	1 cup, 40g	26	•
	Forest Berries	•	¾ cup, 30g	21	•
	Honey Almond	•	⅔ cup, 30g	22	•

★ little or no carbs   ▩ high in saturated fat   ● untested/unknown   Ⓖ GI Symbol partner

GISP	FOOD	GI	SAMPLE SERVING	AVAILABLE CARB (G) PER SERVE	GL PER SERVE
	Sultana Bran varieties				
	Crunch	•	⅔ cup, 45g	32	•
	Original	64	¾ cup, 45g	29	18
	Sanitarium				
	Granola Clusters, all varieties	•	50g	35	•
	Honey Weets	•	30g	24	•
	Light 'n' Tasty, all varieties	68	40g	27–29	19
	Muesli, all varieties	•	50g	29–34	•
	Puffed Wheat	80	30g	21	17
	Skippy corn flakes	93	30g	24	22
	Weet-Bix varieties				
	Bites, all varieties	•	45g	30–34	•
	Hi-Bran	61	2 biscuits, 40g	22	13
	Kids	•	1 biscuit, 15g	10	•
	Lite	•	1 biscuit, 30g	20	•
	Multigrain	•	1 biscuit, 24g	17	•
	Organic	•	2 biscuits, 30g	20	•
	Original	69	2 biscuits, 33g	22	15
	Uncle Tobys				
	Bran Plus	•	45g	12	•
	Cheerios	•	30g	22	•
	Healthwise Heart Wellbeing	•	45g	29	•
	Muesli, Original Swiss Style	62	30g	18	11
	Plus varieties				
	Fibre Lift	•	45g	29	•
	Protein Lift	•	45g	33	•
	Sports Lift	•	45g	32	•
	Quick Oats	82	30g	17	14
	Oatbrits	•	42g	26	•
	Vita Brits	68	33g	23	16
	Weeties	•	30g	20	•

★ little or no carbs　■ high in saturated fat　● untested/unknown　Ⓖ GI Symbol partner

GISP	FOOD	GI	SAMPLE SERVING	AVAILABLE CARB (G) PER SERVE	GL PER SERVE
	**DAIRY PRODUCTS**				
	Milk				
	Regular, whole, 4% fat	27–31	1 cup, 250ml	12	4
	Dairy Farmers	31	250ml	12	4
	Fat-reduced, 1–2% fat	20–30	1 cup, 250ml	15	4
	Farmer's Best with Omega-3, Dairy Farmers	27	250ml	19	5
	HiLo, Pura	20	250ml	14	3
	Lite Start, Pura	30	250ml	13	4
Ⓖ	Lite White, Dairy Farmers	30	250ml	14	4
	Skim, <1% fat	20–34	1 cup, 250ml	12	3
Ⓖ	Dairy Farmers	32	250ml	12	4
	Shape, calcium-enriched	34	250ml	17	6
	Skimmer, Pura	20	250ml	14	3
	Tone, Pura	30	250ml	14	4
	Buttermilk	•	½ cup, 125ml	6	•
	Other milk products				
	Cheese	★	40g	0	•
	Condensed milk, canned, skim	•	½ cup, 125ml	75	•
	Evaporated milk, canned, whole	•	½ cup, 125ml	13	•
	Evaporated milk, canned, reduced fat or skim	•	½ cup, 125ml	14	•
	Powdered milk, whole, dry powder	•	4 tbsp, 30g	11	•
	Powdered milk, skim, dry powder	•	2 tbsp, heaped, 25g	13	•
	Fermented milk drink, Yakult	46	1 bottle, 65ml	12	6
	Fermented milk drink, Yakult Light	36	1 bottle, 65ml	9	3
	Flavoured milk				
	Big M, Chocolate or Strawberry	37	1 carton, 600ml	56–60	22
	Big M, Iced Coffee or Banana	29	1 small carton, 300ml	22	6
	Commercial, full fat milk	34	300ml	28	•
	Full fat, banana, honey & malt flavoured	31	300ml	32	10

★ little or no carbs ■ high in saturated fat ● untested/unknown Ⓖ GI Symbol partner

GISP	FOOD	GI	SAMPLE SERVING	AVAILABLE CARB (G) PER SERVE	GL PER SERVE
	Commercial, low fat, artificially sweetened	24	300ml	18	4
	Commercial, low fat, sugar sweetened	34	300ml	22	7
	Malted milk powder, Nestle, 20 g in full fat milk	45	200ml	24	11
	Malt Milo powder, Nestle, 20 g in full fat milk	37	¾ cup, 200ml	24	9
☺	20g in reduced-fat milk	40	200ml	25	10
☺	20 g in skim milk	46	200ml	24	11
	Masters varieties				
	Iced Coffee light milk	29	1 small carton, 300ml	22	6
	Mocha full fat milk	32	1 carton, 600ml	62	20
	Light, 99% fat free, chocolate or mocha flavour	27	1 carton, 600ml	49–55	14
	Reduced-fat, chocolate or strawberry flavour	35	1 carton, 600ml	49–59	19
	Milo powder, Nestle				
	20 g in full fat milk	33	¾ cup, 200ml	24	8
☺	20 g in reduced fat milk	36	200ml	24	9
☺	20 g in skim milk	39	200ml	24	9
	Nesquik powder, 12g in reduced-fat milk				
	Chocolate flavour	41	¾ cup, 200ml	21	9
	Strawberry flavour	35	¾ cup, 200ml	22	8
	Pauls Good to Go Fruit Smoothie				
	Mango Passionfruit	25	1 cup, 250ml	32	8
	Mixed Berry	30	1 cup, 250ml	32	10
	Strawberry	30	1 cup, 250ml	32	10
	Tropical	25	1 cup, 250ml	32	8
	Rush, low fat, heavenly vanilla malt, ultimate chocolate, wicked latte flavours	26–31	1 bottle, 500ml	27–30	7–9

★ little or no carbs ■ high in saturated fat ● untested/unknown ☺ GI Symbol partner

GISP	FOOD	GI	SAMPLE SERVING	AVAILABLE CARB (G) PER SERVE	GL PER SERVE
	Smoothie varieties				
	Banana	30	1 cup, 250ml	26	8
	Fruit	35	1 cup, 250ml	30	11
	Mango	32	1 cup, 250ml	27	9
	Sustagen varieties				
	Dutch Chocolate	31	1 carton, 250ml	41	13
	Sport drink	43	2 scoops in water, 40g	26	11
	Flavoured soy milk				
	Sanitarium				
	Up & Go, soy & cereal liquid breakfast	43–46	1 cup, 250ml	24–26	11
	Up & Go Vive Banana	44	1 cup, 250ml	26	12
	Up & Go Vive Wild Berry	42	1 cup, 250ml	27	11
	Vitasoy reduced fat chocolate or vanilla	31	1 cup, 250ml	17–19	5–6
	Soy milk				
	Vitasoy, Calci Plus	24	1 cup, 250ml	15	4
	Vitasoy, High Fibre	27	1 cup, 250ml	14	4
	Vitasoy, Lite	17	1 cup, 250ml	8	1
	Vitasoy, Regular	21	1 cup, 250ml	8	2
	Vitasoy, Vitality for Women	18	1 cup, 250ml	9	2
	Yoghurt				
Ⓖ	Brownes Diet No Fat, various flavours	24–40	1 tub, 200g	15	4–6
	Dairy Dream				
	Diet Deli Natural Yoghurt	17	1 tub, 95g	10	2
	Deit Deli Yoghurt with Passionfruit	21	1 tub, 95g	10	2
	Diet Deli Yoghurt with Raspberry	21	1 tub, 95g	9	2
	Dairy Farmers				
	Thick and Creamy 98% Fat Free, various flavours	31–32	1 tub, 170g	26	8
	Light, various flavours	29–33	1 tub, 170g	10–11	3–4

★ little or no carbs   ■ high in saturated fat   ● untested/unknown   Ⓖ GI Symbol partner

GISP	FOOD	GI	SAMPLE SERVING	AVAILABLE CARB (G) PER SERVE	GL PER SERVE
	Jalna varieties				
	Bio Dynamic, bush honey flavour	26	½ cup, 125g	16	4
	Fat Free, natural	19	½ cup, 125g	9	2
	Greek style	12	½ cup, 125g	8	1
	Leben European style	11	½ cup, 125g	9	1
	Premium Blend, creamy vanilla	18	1 tub, 200g	30	5
Ⓖ	Nestle Diet, various flavours	19–21	1 tub, 175g	11	2
	Tamar Valley Greek No Added Sugar Yoghurt, various flavours	21	1 tub, 115g	8–10	2
	Vaalia Kids Probiotic Yoghurt, various flavours	23–27	1 tub, 140g	17	4–5
	Vaalia Light Probiotic Yoghurt French Vanilla	24	1 tub, 150g	11	3
	Vaalia, low fat varieties				
	Lemon crème	43	1 tub, 150g	27	12
	Luscious berries	28	¾ cup, 200g	31	9
	Probiotic Yoghurt Apple Crumble	33	1 tub, 160g	26	9
	Probiotic Yoghurt Apricot Mango Peach	28	1 tub, 100g	15	4
	Probiotic Yoghurt French Vanilla	34	1 tub, 100g	17	6
	Probiotic Yoghurt Vanilla Blueberry	30	1 tub, 100g	16	5
	Passionfruit	32	1 tub, 175g	29	9
	Strawberry	28	1 tub, 175g	28	8
	Yoplait varieties				
	Lite, all flavours	25–37	1 tub, 175g	23–29	8
	Forme, various flavours	16–20	1 tub, 175g	11	2
	Forme Satisfy, various flavours	24–27	1 tub, 170g	11–14	3–4
	Go Gurt, various flavours	39–44	1 tube, 70g	10	4
	Squeezie Pouch, Banana	44	1 pouch, 70g	10	4
	Squeezie Pouch, Blueberry	42	1 pouch, 70g	10	4
	Generic Yoghurt				
	Natural, plain, unflavoured, low fat	14	½ cup, 125g	8	1
	Flavoured	41	1 tub, 200g	24	10

★ **little or no carbs**   ■ **high in saturated fat**   ● **untested/unknown**   Ⓖ **GI Symbol partner**

GISP	FOOD	GI	SAMPLE SERVING	AVAILABLE CARB (G) PER SERVE	GL PER SERVE
	Flavoured, low fat, artificially sweetened	20	½ cup, 125g	7	1
	Custard				
	Homemade, from custard powder, with milk and sugar	43	½ cup, 125ml	14	6
	Low fat, vanilla flavoured, Nestlé	29	½ cup, 125ml	19	5
	Reduced fat, commercial	•	½ cup, 125ml	19	•
	Paul's Trim, vanilla, reduced fat	37	½ cup, 125ml	19	7
	Yogo Choc Rock Chocolate Custard	43	1 tub, 150g	25	11
	Ice-cream, regular, full fat				
	Paddlepop varieties				
	banana, chocolate, rainbow	50–52	1 serve, 68ml	11	6
	Moo, chocolate	48	1 serve, 68ml	13	6
	Moo, strawberry	51	1 serve, 68ml	14	7
	Sara Lee, French vanilla, ultra chocolate flavour	38	2 scoops, 100g	18	7
	Vanilla	47	2 scoops, 100g	21	10
	Ice-cream, Reduced fat				
☺	Chocollo, low-fat, Wendy's	24	1 junior scoop, 80g	11	3
☺	Chocollo, low-fat Wendy's	24	1 junior scoop in waffle cone	55	22
	Light 98% fat free, Vanilla, Bulla	36	2 scoops, 100g	23	8
	Light, low fat, Vanilla, Peter's	46	2 scoops, 100g	30	14
	Low carbohydate, chocolate	32	2 scoops, 100g	4	1
	Low fat, low sugar, Peter's No Sugar Added	•	2 scoops, 100g	8	•
	Vanilla, low fat (1.2% fat), Norco	•	2 scoops, 100g	20	9
	Frozen Yoghurt				
	Vanilla	46	½ cup, 125ml	21	10
	Dairy Desserts				
	Aero Mousse	37	1 tub, 62g	10	4
	Fromage frais	35	1 tub, 125g	15	5

★ little or no carbs   ■ high in saturated fat   ● untested/unknown   ☺ GI Symbol partner

GISP	FOOD	GI	SAMPLE SERVING	AVAILABLE CARB (G) PER SERVE	GL PER SERVE
	Instant pudding, packet mix made with whole milk, chocolate or vanilla	47	100g	16	8
	Nestle Diet varieties				
	Chocolate mousse	31	1 tub, 62g	10	3
	Crème caramel	33	1 tub, 125g	12	4
	Fruche				
	Strawberry fields	•	1 tub, 150g	23	•
	Tropical mango	•	1 tub, 150g	23	•
	Vanilla crème	49	1 tub, 150g	25	12
	Vanilla on mixed berries	49	1 tub, 150g	26	13
	Yoplait Le Rice				
	Apple cinnamon	52	1 tub, 150g	28	15
	Cappucino	46	1 tub, 150g	28	13
	Chocolate	•	1 tub, 150g	27	•
	Classic vanilla	45	1 tub, 150g	27	12
	Mocha	46	1 tub, 150g	29	13
	Smooth caramel	41	1 tub, 150g	29	12
	Forest berries	45	1 tub, 150g	29	13
	Raspberry & white chocolate	51	1 tub, 150g	28	14
	Tropical mango	54	1 tub, 150g	28	15
	DAIRY PRODUCTS – HIGHER GI (MORE THAN 55 OR UNKNOWN)				
	Codensed milk, canned, whole	61	½ cup, 125ml	69	42
	Milk alternatives				
	Oat milk, Vitasoy	69	1 cup, 250ml	23	16
	Rice Milk				
	Australia's Own, low fat	92	1 cup, 250ml	34	31
	Vitasoy rice milk	79	1 cup, 250ml	24	19
	Soy milk, low fat	•	1 cup, 250ml	15	•

★ little or no carbs   ■ high in saturated fat   ● untested/unknown   ☻ GI Symbol partner

GISP	FOOD	GI	SAMPLE SERVING	AVAILABLE CARB (G) PER SERVE	GL PER SERVE
	**FRUIT – LOW GI (LESS THAN OR EQUAL TO 55)**				
	Fresh fruit				
☺	Apple, unpeeled	38	1 medium, 166g	18	7
	Apricot, raw	34	2 regular, 112g	8	3
	Banana	52	1 medium, 120g	24	12
	Blueberries	53	½ cup, 80g	9	5
	Custard apple	54	1 regular, 320g	52	28
	Grapefruit	25	1 medium, 200g	7	2
☺	Grapes	53	⅔ cup, 112g	17	9
	Kiwifruit	53	1 regular, 95g	9	5
	Mango	51	1 regular, 200g	26	13
	Nectarine	43	1 small, 90g	7	3
	Orange	42	1 large, 190g	15	16
	Peach	42	1 medium, 145g	9	4
☺	Pear, unpeeled	38	1 medium, 166g	22	8
	Plum	39	2 regular, 130g	10	4
	Strawberries	40	1 punnet, 250g	8	3
	Dried Fruit				
	Apple	29	4 rings, 25g	16	5
	Apricot	31	10 halves, 35g	16	5
	Dates	39–45	5 regular, 25g	17	7
	Fruit & nut mix	15	¼ cup, 50g	24	4
	Peach	35	3 halves, 40g	16	6
	Pear	43	1 half, 18g	11	5
	Prunes	40	4 regular, 32g	14	6
	Sunmuscats, Sunbeam	53	¼ cup, 50g	32	17
	Tropical fruit & nut mix	49	¼ cup, 50g	14	7
	Canned fruit				
	Apple, canned, Woolworth's Select	42	½ cup, 125g	10	4
	Apricot, canned in natural juice	51	4 halves, 72g	8	4
	Cherries, sour, pitted	41	¼ cup, 130g	12	5

★ little or no carbs ■ high in saturated fat ● untested/unknown ☺ GI Symbol partner

GISP	FOOD	GI	SAMPLE SERVING	AVAILABLE CARB (G) PER SERVE	GL PER SERVE
	Fruit salad, canned in juice	54	1 cup, 263g	26	14
	Grapefruit, ruby red segments canned in juice, Woolworth's Select	47	½ cup, 120g	21	10
	Mandarin, segments, canned in fruit juice	47	½ cup, 130g	18	8
	Orange & grapefruit segments, canned in fruit juice, Woolworth's Select	53	½ cup, 120g	19	10
	Peach, canned in natural juice	45	½ cup, 132g	12	5
	Peaches & grapes, canned in fruit juice, Woolworth's Select	46	½ cup, 120g	12	6
	Peaches & pineapple, canned in fruit juice, Woolworth's Select	45	½ cup, 120g	13	6
	Pear, canned in fruit juice	43	½ cup, 120g	13	6
	Pear, halves, canned in reduced sugar syrup, SPC Lite	25	½ cup, 120g	14	4
	Pineapple, canned in juice, drained, Woolworth's Select	43	1 cup chunks, 200g	20	9
	Pineapple pieces, canned in fruit juice	49	½ cup, 128g	13	6
	Pineapple & papaya pieces, canned in fruit juice, Woolworth's Select	53	½ cup, 120g	17	9

FRUIT – HIGHER GI (MORE THAN 55 OR UNKNOWN)

GISP	FOOD	GI	SAMPLE SERVING	AVAILABLE CARB (G) PER SERVE	GL PER SERVE
Fresh fruit					
	Avocado	★	120g	<1	0
	Blackberries	•	10 regular, 50g	4	•
	Breadfruit	62	¼ cup, 55g	15	9
	Cherries	63	1 cup, 124g	15	9
	Fig, raw, fresh, unpeeled	•	1 large, 64g	5	•
	Fruit salad, fresh, with melon	•	1 cup, 206g	19	•
	Guava	•	1 regular, 90g	3	•
	Honeydew melon	•	1 cup, 180g	12	•
	Lemon	★	1 cup, 40g	0	•
	Lime	★	1 cup, 40g	0	•

★ little or no carbs   ■ high in saturated fat   • untested/unknown   ☉ GI Symbol partner

GISP	FOOD	GI	SAMPLE SERVING	AVAILABLE CARB (G) PER SERVE	GL PER SERVE
	Loquat	●	5 large, 100g	5	●
	Lychees, B3 variety	57	7 regular, 90g	15	9
	Mandarin	●	1 medium, 86g	7	●
	Mulberries	●	1 cup, 148g	6	●
	Nashi pear	●	1 medium, 190g	21	●
	Paw paw	56	1 cup cubed, 148g	10	6
	Persimmon	●	1 medium, 168g	27	●
	Pineapple	59	1 cup, diced 164g	13	8
	Pomegranate, peeled	●	100g	14	●
	Prickly pear, peeled	●	100g	9	●
	Quince, peeled	●	1 medium, 390g	43	●
	Rambutan	●	100g	16	●
	Rockmelon/cantaloupe	88	1 cup diced, 189g	8	7
	Raspberries	★	100g	7	●
	Rhubarb	★	125g	0	0
	Tamarillo, peeled	●	100g	3	●
	Tangelo, peeled	●	100g	8	●
	Watermelon	78	100g	3	2
	Canned fruit				
	Apricot, canned in light syrup	64	4 halves, 90g	12	8
	Lychees, canned in syrup, drained	79	7 regular, 90g	16	13
	Peach, canned in light syrup	57	½ cup, 132g	17	10
	Dried Fruit				
	Cranberries, sweetened	64	2 tbsp, 25g	16	10
	Currants	●	2 tbsp, 24g	16	●
	Fig	61	2 regular, 20g 100g	21 55	13
	Mixed fruit	●	100g	65	●
	Raisins	61	1½ tbsp, 20g	16	10
	Sultanas	56	1½ tbsp, 20g	15	8

★ little or no carbs   ■ high in saturated fat   ● untested/unknown   Ⓖ GI Symbol partner

GISP	FOOD	GI	SAMPLE SERVING	AVAILABLE CARB (G) PER SERVE	GL PER SERVE
	LEGUMES				
	Baked beans				
	Canned In Tomato Sauce	52	½ cup, 150g	18	9
	Heinz varieties, canned				
	Barbecue sauce	47	1 sml can, 220g	34	16
	Cheesy tomato sauce	44	1 sml can, 220g	28	12
	Ham sauce	53	1 sml can, 220g	31	16
	Mild curry sauce	49	1 sml can, 220g	34	17
	Sweet chilli sauce	46	1 sml can, 220g	33	15
	Tomato sauce	49	1 sml can, 220g	30	15
	Black-eyed beans				
	Dried, uncooked	•	100g	60	•
	Soaked, boiled	42	½ cup, 75g	17	7
	Borlotti beans				
	Dried, uncooked	•	100g	35	•
	Canned, drained, Edgell	41	½ cup, 75g	12	5
	Butter beans				
	Soaked, boiled	26	½ cup, 75g	8	2
	Canned, drained, Edgell	36	½ cup, 80g	11	4
	Cannellini beans				
	Cooked from dried beans	•	½ cup, 86g	12	•
	Canned, drained, Edgell	31	½ cup, 128g	15	5
	Chickpeas				
	Canned, drained	40	½ cup, 80g	11	4
	Canned, drained, Edgell	38	1 can, 75g	13	5
	Hommus, Chris' Traditional	22	2 tbsp, 40g	3	1
	Four bean mix				
	Canned, drained, Edgell	37	1 can, 75g	12	4
	Haricot/Navy bean				
	Dried, uncooked	•	100g	35	•
	Boiled	33	½ cup, 88g	12	4

★ little or no carbs   ■ high in saturated fat   ● untested/unknown   ⓖ GI Symbol partner

GISP	FOOD	GI	SAMPLE SERVING	AVAILABLE CARB (G) PER SERVE	GL PER SERVE
	Lentils				
	Brown, canned	42	½ cup, 80g	13	5
	Green, dried, boiled	30	⅔ cup, 125g	17	5
	Green, canned	48	⅔ cup, 135g	17	8
	Red, dried, boiled	26	⅔ cup, 125g	18	5
	Red, dried, split, boiled 25 min	21	125g	15	3
	Dhal	●	1 cup, 195g	29	●
	Mung beans				
	Boiled	39	⅔ cup, 127g	15	4
	Red kidney beans				
	Dried, uncooked	●	100g	36	●
	Dried, boiled	51	100g	9	5
	Canned, drained, Edgell	36	1 can, 75g	11	4
	Pinto beans				
	Refried, canned, Casa Fiesta	38	½ cup, 115g	20	8
	Steamed	33	½ cup, 150g	23	8
	Snake beans				
	Snake beans	★	70g	0	●
	Soup Mix				
	Dry, standard	●	100g	50	●
	Dry, Italian	●	100g	40	●
	Soy beans				
	Dried, uncooked	●	100g	13	●
	Dried, boiled	18	1 cup, 170g	4	1
	Canned, drained, Edgell	14	½ cup, 100g	3	0
	Split peas				
	Dried, uncooked, yellow/green	●	¼ cup, 53g	25	●
	Dried, boiled, yellow/green	25	1 cup, 180g	13	3

★ little or no carbs ■ high in saturated fat ● untested/unknown Ⓖ GI Symbol partner

GISP	FOOD	GI	SAMPLE SERVING	AVAILABLE CARB (G) PER SERVE	GL PER SERVE
	MEAT, SEAFOOD & PROTEIN				
	Bacon	★ ■	50g	0	•
	Beef, lean	★	120g	0	•
	Brawn	★ ■	75g	0	•
	Calamari rings, squid, not battered or crumbed	★	70g	0	•
	Chicken, no skin	★	110g	0	•
	Duck	★ ■	140g	0	•
	Eggs	★ ■	120g	0	•
	Fish	★	120g	0	•
	Ham, lean	★	24g	0	•
	Lamb	★	120g	0	•
	Liver Sausage	★ ■	30g	0	•
	Liverwurst	★ ■	30g	0	•
	Oysters, natural, plain	★	85g	0	•
	Pork, lean	★	120g	0	•
	Prawns	★	150g	0	•
	Salami	★ ■	120g	0	•
	Salmon, fresh or canned in water or brine	★	150g	0	•
	Sardines	★	60g	0	•
	Sausages, fried	28 ■	100g	3	1
	Scallops, natural, plain	★	160g	0	•
	Shellfish	★	120g	0	•
	Steak, lean	★	120g	0	•
	Tofu, bean curd, plain, unsweetened	★	100g	0	•
	Trout, fresh or frozen	★	63g	0	•
	Tuna, fresh or canned in water or brine	★	120g	0	•
	Turkey, lean	★	140g	0	•
	Veal	★	120g	0	•

★ little or no carbs   ■ high in saturated fat   ● untested/unknown   Ⓖ GI Symbol partner

GISP	FOOD	GI	SAMPLE SERVING	AVAILABLE CARB (G) PER SERVE	GL PER SERVE
	RICE, PASTA, NOODLES & GRAINS – LOW GI (LESS THAN OR EQUAL TO 55)				
	Barley				
	Pearl, raw	•	2 tbsp, 32g	15	•
	Pearl, boiled	25	1 cup, 190g	40	10
	Bulgur (burghul)				
	Raw	•	2 tbsp, 25g	15	•
	Boiled	•	1 cup, 265g	46	•
	Soaked in water	48	100g	28	13
	Buckwheat				
	Groats, raw	•	2 tbsp, 30g	21	•
	Groats, boiled	54	1 cup, 180g	34	18
	Couscous				
Ⓖ	Blu Gourmet pearl couscous, cooked	52	½ cup	19	10
	Rice				
	Doongara rice, CleverRice, SunRice	53	1 cup, 170g	44	23
	Long-grain rice, white, boiled 15 min, Mahatma	50	1 cup, 170g	46	23
	Noodles				
	Instant 2-minute noodles, Maggi	52	1 pkt, 380g	56	29
	Mung bean noodles, Lungkow bean thread, dried, boiled	39	1 cup, 180g	45	18
	Rice noodles, fresh, boiled	40	1 cup, 180g	39	16
	Soba noodles, instant, served in soup	46	1 cup, 180g	49	23
	Quinoa				
	Dry	•	¼ cup, 43g	27	•
	Boiled, Nature First Organic	53	⅓ cup, 62g	13	7
	Semolina				
	Raw	•	2 tbsp, 26g	17	•
	Cooked	55	1 cup, 245g	17	10

★ little or no carbs ■ high in saturated fat ● untested/unknown Ⓖ GI Symbol partner

GISP	FOOD	GI	SAMPLE SERVING	AVAILABLE CARB (G) PER SERVE	GL PER SERVE
	Pasta				
	Capellini	45	1 cup, 150g	45	20
	Fettuccine, egg	40	1 cup, 180g	46	18
	Fusilli twists, tricolour	51	1 cup, 150g	42	21
	Lasagne, beef, commercial	47	200g	30	14
	Latina Fresh Pasta				
	Agnolotti, ricotta & spinach	47	½ pkt, 280g	83	39
	Fettuccine, egg	54	½ pkt, 360g	92	50
	Lasagne sheets	49	1 regular, 47g	23	11
	Ravioli, beef	43	½ pkt, 315g	70	30
	Ravioli, chicken & garlic	44	½ pkt, 279g	76	33
	Ravioli, wholegrain, ricotta & spinach	39	½ pkt, 220g	58	23
	Tortellini, mixed veal	48	½ pkt, 305g	80	38
	Vetta varieties				
Ⓖ	Lasagne sheets	53	1 regular, 19g	13	7
Ⓖ	Macaroni, boiled 8–10 min	49	1 cup, 150g	40	20
Ⓖ	Spaghetti, boiled 8–10 min	49	1 cup, 180g	48	24
	Macaroni	47	1 cup, 150g	40	19
	Spaghetti	44	1 cup, 180g	48	21
	Spaghetti, protein-enriched	27	1 cup, 180g	14	4
	Spaghetti, wholemeal	42	1 cup, 180g	42	18
	Spirali, white, durum wheat	43	1 cup, 150g	44	19
	Star Pastina, white, boiled 5 min	38	1 cup, 150g	48	18
	Vermicelli	35	1 cup, 180g	48	17
	White, boiled	•	1 cup, 140g	35	•
	White, dry	•	⅓ cup, 45g	30	•
	Instant pasta				
	Pasta & sauce, prepared, Woolworth's Select	48–57	¼ pkt, 110g	20–23	10–12
	Gluten-free pasta				
	Rice pasta, Freedom Foods	51	1 cup, 180g	47	24

★ little or no carbs ■ high in saturated fat ● untested/unknown Ⓖ GI Symbol partner

GISP	FOOD	GI	SAMPLE SERVING	AVAILABLE CARB (G) PER SERVE	GL PER SERVE
RICE, PASTA, NOODLES & GRAINS – HIGHER GI (MORE THAN 55 OR UNKNOWN)					
	Cornmeal/Polenta				
	Raw	•	2 tbsp, 20g	14	•
	Boiled	68	1 cup, 250g	22	15
	Couscous				
	Raw	•	¼ cup, 40g	30	•
	Cooked, soaked	65	1 cup, 160g	15	10
	Flours				
	Wheat, white	•	1 tbsp, 13g	8	•
	Wheat, wholemeal	•	1 tbsp, 13g	8	•
	Millet, raw	•	100g	63	•
	Millet, boiled	71	100g	23	16
	Noodles				
	Buckwheat noodles	59	180g	42	25
	Instant 2-Minute Noodles, Maggi, 99% fat free	67	1 pkt, 380g	56	38
	Rice vermicelli, dried, boiled	58	¼ pkt, 250g	50	29
	Rice pasta, brown, boiled	92	1 cup, 180g	38	35
	Asian, shelf stable noodles, e.g. Hokkein, Singapore	•	½ pkt, 110g	35	•
	Udon, plain	62	½ pkt, 200g	50	31
	Pasta				
	Gnocchi, cooked	68	100g	29	20
	Macaroni & cheese, prepared, Kraft	64	302g	76	49
	Gluten-free pasta				
	Corn pasta, Orgran	78	1 cup, 180g	42	33
	Rice and maize pasta, Ris'O'Mais, Orgran	76	1 cup, 180g	49	37
	Spaghetti, canned in tomato sauce, Orgran	68	1 can, 220g	27	18

★ little or no carbs   ■ high in saturated fat   ● untested/unknown   Ⓖ GI Symbol partner

GISP	FOOD	GI	SAMPLE SERVING	AVAILABLE CARB (G) PER SERVE	GL PER SERVE
	Rice				
	Raw	●	¼ cup, 50g	40	●
	Boiled	●	1 cup, 170g	45	●
	Arborio/risotto rice, boiled, SunRice	69	1 cup, 170g	49	34
	Basmati rice, white, boiled	58	1 cup, 170g	47	27
	Basmati White Rice, SunRice, boiled	59	1 cup, 170g	44	26
	Broken Rice, Thai, white, cooked in rice cooker	86	1 cup, 170g	49	42
	Brown rice, boiled/pelde	86	1 cup, 170g	43	37
	Calrose rice, brown, medium-grain, boiled	76	1 cup, 170g	45	34
	Calrose rice, white, medium-grain, boiled	87	1 cup, 170g	48	42
	Glutinous rice, white, cooked in rice cooker	98	½ cup, 170g	36	35
	Instant rice, white, cooked 6 min with water	87	1 cup, 170g	48	42
	Japanese-style sushi rice, SunRice	73	1 cup, 170g	46	34
	Jasmine fragrant rice, SunRice	89	1 cup, 170g	45	40
	Koshihikari White Rice, RunRice, boiled	61	1 cup, 170g	43	26
	Medium-Grain, Brown SunRice	59	1 cup, 170g	49	29
	Parboiled rice, Pelde, Sungold	87	1 cup, 170g	49	43
	Sri Lankan Red Rice, boiled	59	1 cup, 170g	45	27
	Sunbrown Quick rice, Ricegrowers, boiled	80	1 cup, 170g	43	34
	Uncle Ben's Express Microwave Basmati Rice	63	100g	30	19
	Uncle Ben's Microwave Long Grain Rice	59	100g	31	18
	White long-grain rice, Premium, SunRice	59	1 cup, 170g	45	27
	Wild rice, boiled	57	½ cup, 75g	15	9

★ little or no carbs   ■ high in saturated fat   ● untested/unknown   Ⓖ GI Symbol partner

GISP	FOOD	GI	SAMPLE SERVING	AVAILABLE CARB (G) PER SERVE	GL PER SERVE
	Spelt				
	Dry	•	100g	59	•
	Cooked	•	100g	23	•
	Wheat				
	Wheat bran, unprocessed	•	100g	16	•
	Wheatgerm	•	100g	30	•

★ little or no carbs ■ high in saturated fat ● untested/unknown Ⓖ GI Symbol partner

GISP	FOOD	GI	SAMPLE SERVING	AVAILABLE CARB (G) PER SERVE	GL PER SERVE
	SNACKFOODS & TREATS – LOW GI (LESS THAN OR EQUAL TO 55)				
	Cakes & pastries				
	Banana cake, homemade	51	1 slice, 80g	38	19
	Bavarian, chocolate honeycomb, Sara Lee Lite	31	¼ cake, 93g	25	8
	Carrot cake, commercially made	38	1 sml slice, 50g	19	7
	Chocolate brownies	42	1 serve, 56g	30	13
	Chocolate cake, pkt mix, with frosting, Betty Crocker	38	1 slice, 110g	52	20
	Chocolate mud cake	43	1 slice, 100g	54	29
	Chocolate crackles	43	1 serve, 12g	12	5
	Crumble, apple berry, commercially made	41	1 slice, 165g	34	14
	Danish, apple & peach, Sara Lee Lite	50	⅛ pkt, 67g	29	15
	Egg Tart, Chinese style	45	1 serve, 60g	21	9
	Fruit cake, commercial, Big Sister	53	1 slice, 50g	28	15
	Pavlova, prepared with fresh cream, strawberries, banana and passionfruit	49	1 slice, 120g	33	16
	Pound cake	54	1 sml slice, 50g	23	12
	Sponge cake, plain, unfilled	46	1 slice, 25g	14	6
	Vanilla cake, from pkt mix with frosting, Betty Crocker	42	1 slice, 65g	31	13
	Savoury snacks				
	Chickpea chips, Freedom Foods	44	⅓ pkt, 50g	25	11
	Corn chips	42	1 pkt, 50g	26	11
	Grain Waves Wholegrain chips, original, Smith's	51	1 pkt, 40g	25	13
	Confectionery				
	Chocolate	42–49	4 sml squares, 24g	15	7
	Chocolate coated almonds	21	5–6 almonds, 30g	8	2
	Chocolate, dark, Dove	23	4 sml squares, 24g	13	3
	Chocolate, fructose sweetened	20	4 sml squares, 24g	15	3
	Chocolate, white, Milky Bar, Nestle	44	1 fun size, 15g	8	4

★ little or no carbs   ■ high in saturated fat   ● untested/unknown   Ⓖ GI Symbol partner

GISP	FOOD	GI	SAMPLE SERVING	AVAILABLE CARB (G) PER SERVE	GL PER SERVE
	Jelly, diet, made from crystals with water	★	½ cup, 120g	0	●
	Jelly, made from commercial jelly crystals	53	½ cup, 120g	19	10
	M&M's, peanut, Mars	33	1 fun size, 14g	8	3
	Milo bar, Nestle	40	1 serve, 21g	15	6
	Rum balls, Woolworth's	50	1 serve, 25g	14	7
	Snickers bar, Mars	41	1 fun size, 22g	13	5
	Twix bar, Mars	44	1 fun size, 16g	10	4
	Yummiees jelly lollies, Allseps	43	4 lollies, 15g	5	2
Muffins					
	Apple, homemade	46	1 regular, 60g	29	13
	Apple blueberry, Sara Lee	49	1 regular, 60g	25	12
	Apple, oat, sultana	54	1 regular, 50g	26	14
	Blueberry, Sara Lee	50	1 regular, 60g	31	16
	Chocolate	53	1 regular, 60g	30	16
	Choc-butterscotch	53	1 regular, 50g	28	15
	Choc-chip, Sara Lee	52	1 regular, 60g	32	17
	Double chocolate	46	1 regular, 60g	34	16
Nuts					
	Almonds	●	½ cup, 75g	3	●
	Cashews	22	½ cup, 100g	26	6
	Chestnut, roasted	●	5 kernels, 100g	34	●
	Dried fruit & nut mix, commercial	32	¼ cup, 50g	22	7
	Macadamia	●	½ cup, 75g	3	●
	Mixed nuts, roasted, salted	24	½ cup, 100g	25	6
	Peanut, dry roasted	23	½ cup, 100g	9	2
	Pecan	10	½ cup, 100g	5	1
	Pine nut	●	½ cup, 100g	5	●
	Sesame seeds	★	12g	0	●
	Walnut	●	½ cup, 53g	<0.5	●
Snack bars					
	Bakers Delight, Fit2Go Bars				

★ little or no carbs ■ high in saturated fat ● untested/unknown Ⓖ GI Symbol partner

GISP	FOOD	GI	SAMPLE SERVING	AVAILABLE CARB (G) PER SERVE	GL PER SERVE
	Cranberry & Nuts bar	51	1 bar, 77g	25	13
	Fruit & Cinnamon bar	53	1 bar, 77g	28	15
	Be Natural Four Bars				
	Coconut, Apricot, Oats & Chia	41	1 bar, 32g	14	6
	Currant, Berry, Oats & Pepita	48	1 bar, 32g	15	7
	Be Natural Nut Bars				
	Almond Apricot	44	1 bar, 40g	18	8
	Fruit and Nut	38	1 bar, 50g	18	7
	Nut Delight	29	1 bar, 40g	11	3
	Be Natural Trail Bars				
	Dark Chocolate & Nut	55	1 bar, 32g	19	11
	Honey Nut	54	1 bar, 32g	19	10
	Carman's				
	Apricot & Almond Muesli Bar	51	1 bar, 45g	23	12
	Apricot Muesli Bites	54	20g	12	6
	Classic Fruit Muesli Bar	53	1 bar, 45g	26	14
	Classic Fruit Muesli Bites	52	20g	12	6
	Dark Chocolate, Cranberry & Almond Bar	53	1 bar, 35g	19	10
	Original Fruit-Free Muesli Bar	55	1 bar, 45g	24	13
	Yoghurt, Apricot & Almond Bar	44	1 bar, 35g	18	8
	Freedom Foods				
	Hi-Lite breakfast bar	53	1 bar, 35g	21	11
	Omega Bar, gluten-free, seed & nut	21	1 bar, 40g	17	4
	Superberry breakfast bar	54	1 bar, 35g	20	11
	Healtheries Simple Snack Bar				
	Apricot & yoghurt	40	1 bar, 45g	23	9
	Berry & yoghurt	51	1 bar, 45g	24	12
	Chocolate	35	1 bar, 45g	25	9
	Ironman PR bar, chocolate	39	1 bar, 65g	26	10
	Kellogg's Crunch Nut Nutty				
	Mixed Nut Bar	36	1 bar, 30g	14	5
	Peanut Bar	34	1 bar, 30g	14	5

★ little or no carbs   ■ high in saturated fat   ● untested/unknown   ⓖ GI Symbol partner

GISP	FOOD	GI	SAMPLE SERVING	AVAILABLE CARB (G) PER SERVE	GL PER SERVE
	Kellogg's K-Time Twists varieties				
	Apple & Cinnamon	51	1 bar, 37g	24	12
	Raspberry & Apple	55	1 bar, 37g	24	13
	Strawberry & Blueberry	45	1 bar, 37g	24	11
	Strawberry & Yoghurt	47	1 bar, 37g	24	11
	Mother Earth Baked Fruit Stick, apricot-filled	50	1 bar, 19g	13	7
	Sunripe School Straps,				
☻	Blackberry sour buzz	35	1 bar, 15g	10	4
☻	Strawberry & wildberry	40	1 bar, 15g	10	4
	Trim Low-GI protein snack bar, Aussie Bodies				
	Berryliscious	46	1 bar, 50g	15	7
	Chocorama	31	1 bar, 50g	14	4
	Uncle Tobys, muesli bar varieties				
☻	Chewy, forest fruit	48	1 bar, 31g	20	10
☻	Chewy, white choc chip	54	1 bar, 31g	20	11
☻	Chewy, choc chip	54	1 bar, 31g	20	11
☻	Crunchy, apricot	54	1 bar, 31g	20	11
☻	Crunchy, forest fruit	48	1 bar, 31g	20	10
☻	Crunchy, choc chip	54	1 bar, 31g	20	11

SNACKFOODS & TREATS – HIGHER GI (MORE THAN 55 OR UNKNOWN)

Cakes & Pastries

GISP	FOOD	GI	SAMPLE SERVING	AVAILABLE CARB (G) PER SERVE	GL PER SERVE
	Angel food cake	67	1 sml piece, 57g	31	21
	Chinese Moon Cakes	56	1 cake, 80g	50	28
	Chinese Pineapple Bun	65	1 bun, 62g	34	22
	Cupcake, strawberry iced	73	1 serve, 38g	26	19
	Fruit mince pies, Mr Kipling	58	1 serve, 59g	35	20
	Glutinous Rice Ball	61	1 serve, 220g	95	58
	Lamington	87	1 serve, 50g	29	25
	Puff pastry	56	100g	40	22
	Red Bean Dessert	75	1 serve, 200g	38	29

★ little or no carbs   ■ high in saturated fat   ● untested/unknown   ☻ GI Symbol partner

GISP	FOOD	GI	SAMPLE SERVING	AVAILABLE CARB (G) PER SERVE	GL PER SERVE
	Savoury snacks				
	Burger Rings	90	1 pkt, 50g	29	26
	Chips, potato	57	1 mini pkt, 25g	12	7
	Poppin Microwave Popcorn varieties, Green's Foods				
	Butter	62	1 pkt, 100g	50	31
	Lite	67	1 pkt, 85g	48	32
	plain	72	1 cup, 9g	5	4
	Prawn cracker	•	1 pkt, 50g	33	•
	Pretzels	•	1 cup, 42g	27	•
	Pretzels, oven-baked, traditional wheat flavour, Parkers	84	10 pretzels, 19g	15	13
	Rice crackers	91	11 crackers, 19g	15	14
	Twisties, Smith's	74	1 pkt, 30g	19	14
	Confectionery				
	Gummi confectionery	94	6 pieces, 24g	15	14
	Jelly beans	78	10–15 lollies, 30g	28	22
	Licorice, soft	78	1 stick, 12g	9	7
	Life Savers, peppermint candy, Nestle	70	1 pkt, 22g	21	15
	Mars Bar, Mars	62	1 fun size, 22g	16	10
	Marshmallows, plain, pink & white	62	4 small, 20g	16	10
	Milky Way bar, Mars	62	1 fun size, 14g	10	6
	Skittles, fruit candies, Mars	70	1 fun size, 25g	23	16
	Muffins				
	Apricot, coconut & honey	60	1 regular, 50g	26	16
	Banana, oat & honey	65	1 regular, 50g	26	17
	Blueberry, commercially made	59	1 regular, 57g	29	17
	Bran, commercially made	60	1 regular, 57g	24	14
	Carrot, commercially made	62	1 regular, 57g	32	20
	Oatmeal, from pkt mix	69	1 regular, 50g	35	24
	Snack bars				
	Roll-Ups, processed fruit snack, Uncle Tobys	99	1 serve, 15g	11	11

★ little or no carbs   ■ high in saturated fat   ● untested/unknown   ☻ GI Symbol partner

GISP	FOOD	GI	SAMPLE SERVING	AVAILABLE CARB (G) PER SERVE	GL PER SERVE
	SPREADS & SWEETENERS – LOW GI (LESS THAN OR EQUAL TO 55)				
	Agave Nectar, premium, Sweet Cactus Farms	19	1 tsp, 5g	3	1
	Divine Date spread, Buderim Ginger	29	1 tbsp, 25g	16	5
Ⓖ	Fruisana Fructose, pure	19	1 sachet, 10g	10	2
	Ginger, sucrose free, Buderim Ginger	10	4 pieces, 20g	15	2
	Honey				
	Ironbark	48	2 tsp, 14g	12	6
	Red gum	53	2 tsp, 14g	12	6
	Stringybark	44	2 tsp, 14g	12	5
	Yapunya	52	2 tsp, 14g	12	6
	Yellowbox	35	2 tsp, 14g	12	4
Ⓖ	LoGiCane, low GI cane sugar	50	1 tsp, 4g	4	2
	Maple syrup, pure	54	1 tbsp, 27g	18	10
	Marmalade, ginger, Buderim Ginger	50	1 tbsp, 18g	13	7
	Marmalade, orange	55	2 tbsp, 25g	16	9
	Nutella, hazelnut spread, Ferrero	25	2 tsp, 10g	5	1
	Strawberry jam, regular	51	1 tbsp, 25g	17	9
	St Dalfour				
	Black Cherry Jam	50	1 tbsp, 25g	13	6
	Blackberry Jam	54	1 tbsp, 25g	13	7
	Golden Peach Jam	50	1 tbsp, 25g	13	7
	Gourmet Pear Jam	53	1 tbsp, 25g	13	7
	Mirabelle Plum Jam	54	1 tbsp, 25g	13	7
	Orange Marmalade	54	1 tbsp, 25g	14	8
	Pineapple Mango Jam	55	1 tbsp, 25g	13	7
	Raspberry & Pomegranate Jam	55	1 tbsp, 25g	14	8
	Red Raspberry Jam	55	1 tbsp, 25g	14	8
	Royal Fig Jam	51	1 tbsp, 25g	13	6
	Strawberry Jam	52	1 tbsp, 25g	13	7

★ little or no carbs   ■ high in saturated fat   ● untested/unknown   Ⓖ GI Symbol partner

GISP	FOOD	GI	SAMPLE SERVING	AVAILABLE CARB (G) PER SERVE	GL PER SERVE
	Thick Apricot Jam	54	1 tbsp, 25g	13	7
	Wild Blueberry Jam	52	1 tbsp, 25g	13	7
Ⓖ	Sweetaddin	19	2 tsp, 10g	10	2
SPREADS & SWEETENERS – HIGHER GI (MORE THAN 55 OR UNKNOWN)					
	Golden syrup	63	2 tsp, 14g	10	6
	Honey	•	2 tsp, 14g	12	•
	Blended	64	2 tsp, 14g	12	8
	Salvation Jane	64	2 tsp, 14g	12	8
	Maple-flavoured syrup, Cottees	68	1 tbsp, 20g	11	7
	Sugar	68	1 tsp, 5g	5	3
	Treacle	68	3 tsp, 20g	13	9
	Vinegar	★	1 tsp, 5ml	0	•

★ little or no carbs ■ high in saturated fat ● untested/unknown Ⓖ GI Symbol partner

GISP	FOOD	GI	SAMPLE SERVING	AVAILABLE CARB (G) PER SERVE	GL PER SERVE
	TAKEAWAY & PRE-PREPARED MEALS				
	— LOW GI (LESS THAN OR EQUAL TO 55)				
	Burrito, corn tortilla, refried beans & tomato salsa	39	1 serve, 100g	23	9
	Cannelloni, spinach & ricotta, prepared convenience meal	15	1 serve, 300g	54	8
	Chicken nuggets, frozen, reheated in microwave 5 min	46	6 nuggets, 100g	16	7
	Dosai, served with chutney	55	1 serve, 150g	39	21
	Fajitas, chicken	42	1 serve, 300g	42	18
	Fish fingers	38	4 fingers, 100g	18	7
	Lasagne, beef, commercially made	47	1 serve, 300g	35	16
	Meat pie	45	1 regular, 175g	41	18
	Party pies, beef, commercial	45	1 regular, 38g	10	5
	Moussaka, lamb, prepared convenience meal	35	1 serve, 300g	27	9
	Pizza Hut varieties				
	Supreme, thin & crispy,	30	1 slice, 71g	17	5
	Super Supreme, pan	36	1 slice, 94	23	8
	Veggie Supreme, thin & crispy	49	1 slice, 63g	16	8
	Generic				
	Pork Puff, Asian, BBQ pork, commercial	55	1 portion, 54g	17	9
	Singapore Fried Vermicelli Noodles	54	1 serve, 300g	45	24
	Spaghetti Bolognaise	52	1 serve, 360g	48	25
	Spring Roll	50	1 roll, 80g	45	24
	Sushi, salmon	48	2 med pieces, 100g	14	7
☺	Sushi, tofu and pickled radish nori roll with brown rice. Keepin it Fresh	45	1 roll, 200g	42	19
	Vine leaves, stuffed with rice & lamb, served with tomato sauce	30	1 serve, 100g	15	5

★ little or no carbs ■ high in saturated fat ● untested/unknown ☺ GI Symbol partner

GISP	FOOD	GI	SAMPLE SERVING	AVAILABLE CARB (G) PER SERVE	GL PER SERVE
	Pasta sauce, Latina Fresh varieties				
	Bolognese sauce	24	½ tub, 212g	15	4
	Creamy Sun dried tomato	19	½ tub, 212g	18	3
	Italian tomato & garlic	40	½ tub, 212g	14	6
	Mediterranean sauce	40	½ tub, 212g	10	4
	Soups				
	Barley & vegetable	41	1 cup, 250ml	28	11
	Carrot, canned	35	1 cup, 250ml	13	5
	Lentil, canned	44	1 cup, 250ml	21	9
	Tomato, canned	45	1 cup, 250ml	17	8
	**TAKEAWAY & PRE-PREPARED MEALS** **— HIGHER GI (MORE THAN 55 OR UNKNOWN)**				
	Baked potato with baked beans	62	1 serve, 140g	37	23
	Battered fish, commercial	●	1 serve, 100g	14	●
	Chiko roll	●	1 serve, 100g	26	●
	Chips, takeaway	●	1 serve, 100g	26	●
	Crumbed calamari	●	1 serve, 100g	16	●
	Dim sim, commercial, deep fried	●	1 serve, 100g	27	●
	French fries, frozen, reheated in microwave	75	1 serve, 150g	29	22
	Fried chicken, e.g. KFC	●	1 serve, 100g	6	●
	Fried Fritter	69	1 roll, 200g	35	24
	Fried rice in Yangzhou-style	80	1 serve, 300g	69	55
	Fried rice noodles with sliced beef	66	1 serve, 300g	60	40
	Pork Bun, Asian, commercial	69	1 bun, 60g	25	17
	Potato scallop	●	1 serve, 100g	27	●
	Sausages and mash, prepared, convenience meal	61	1 serve, 500g	67	41
	Shepherds pie	66	1 serve, 500g	74	49
	Steak, mashed potato & mixed vegetables, homemade	66	1 serve, 360g	53	35
	Steamed Vermicelli roll	90	1 roll, 190g	40	36

★ little or no carbs   ■ high in saturated fat   ● untested/unknown   Ⓖ GI Symbol partner

GISP	FOOD	GI	SAMPLE SERVING	AVAILABLE CARB (G) PER SERVE	GL PER SERVE
	Steamed Glutinous Rice roll	89	1 roll, 94g	43	39
	Sticky Rice in Lotus Leaf	83	1 serve, 300g	89	74
	Taco shells, cornmeal-based, baked	68	2 regular, 26g	14	10
	Soups				
	Chicken & mushroom	58	1 cup, 250ml	18	10
	Clear consommé, chicken or vegetable	★	1 cup, 205ml	0	•
	Green pea, canned	66	1 cup, 250ml	41	27
	Pumpkin, creamy, Heinz Very Special	76	1 cup, 290ml	29	22
	Spicy Thai instant soup, low fat	56	1 cup, 250ml	31	17
	Split pea, canned	60	1 cup, 250ml	27	16
	Vegetable	60	1 cup, 250ml	18	11

★ little or no carbs ■ high in saturated fat ● untested/unknown Ⓖ GI Symbol partner

GISP	FOOD	GI	SAMPLE SERVING	AVAILABLE CARB (G) PER SERVE	GL PER SERVE
	**STARCHY VEGETABLES – LOW GI (LESS THAN OR EQUAL TO 55)**				
	Carrot	39	1 medium, 61g	3	1
	Carrot juice	43	1 cup, 250ml	14	6
	Cassava, peeled, diced, boiled	46	1 cup, 140g	42	19
	Corn on cob	48	1 medium, 77g	16	8
	Corn, loose kernels	48	½ cup, 87g	17	8
	Corn, canned	46	½ cup, 88g	16	7
	Corn, creamed, canned	●	⅓ can, 86g	14	●
	Parsnip, boiled	52	1 cup, 100g	10	5
	Parsnip, baked	●	100g	12	●
	Peas, green, fresh or frozen, boiled	51	½ cup, 80g	6	3
	Peas, canned	●	100g	9	●
☺	Potato, Carisma, unpeeled, boiled 4 min (or until al dente), Coles	55	1 medium, 125g	16	9
	Potato, Nadine, baked	54	150g	20	11
	Potato, Nadine, boiled	49	150g	20	10
	Pumpkin, raw	●	1 cup, 100g	6	●
	Pumpkin, baked	●	1 cup, 100g	8	●
	Pumpkin, butternut, boiled, mashed	51	2 scoops, 100g	8	4
	Taro	54	½ cup, 100g	25	14
	Yam, peeled, boiled	54	1 cup, 100g	25	14
	**STARCHY VEGETABLES – HIGHER GI (MORE THAN 55 OR UNKNOWN)**				
	Beetroot, fresh, boiled	●	1 whole, 82g	7	●
	Beetroot, canned	64	4 slices, 32g	3	2
	Mixed vegetables, frozen e.g., peas, carrot, swede, beans, sweet corn	●	½ cup	11	●
	Potato, baked, peeled, without oil	●	2 med chunks, 100g	20	●
	Potato, baked, jacket, in foil, without oil	●	1 large, 200g	28	●
	Potato, Nadine, cooked in microwave	57	150g	20	11

★ little or no carbs   ■ high in saturated fat   ● untested/unknown   ☺ GI Symbol partner

GISP	FOOD	GI	SAMPLE SERVING	AVAILABLE CARB (G) PER SERVE	GL PER SERVE
	Potato chips, frozen, oven heat	●	15–20 chips, 100g	45	●
	Potato, Desiree, peeled, boiled 35 min	101	1 medium, 150g	17	17
	Potato Gems	●	12 gems	31	●
	Potato, Hash Browns	●	1 patty	12	●
	Potato, mashed, instant, Edgell	86	¼ pkt, 150g	20	17
	Potato, mashed potato, with butter and milk	●	½ cup, 100g	11	●
	Potato, new	78	2 small, 140g	18	14
	Potato, new, canned, microwaved	65	3–4 small, 120g	17	11
	Potato, Nicola, unpeeled, boiled whole 15 min	58	3 small, 150g	16	9
	Potato, Pontiac, peeled, boiled 15 min, mashed	91	½ cup, 150g	20	18
	Potato Pontiac, peeled, boiled whole 30–35 min	72	1 medium, 150g	18	13
	Potato Pontiac, peeled, microwaved 7 min	79	1 medium, 150g	18	14
	Potato, Sebago, peeled, boiled 35 min	87	1 medium, 150g	17	15
	Potato, wedges, with skin, frozen, oven heat	●	2 large, 50g	44	●
	Pumpkin, boiled	66	1 cup, 100g	7	5
	Swede, diced	72	1 cup, 170g	7	5
	Sweet potato, orange, peeled, cut into pieces, boiled 8 min	61	100g	15	9
	Sweet potato, purple skin, white flesh raw, diced	●	100g	14	●
	Sweet potato, purple skin white flesh, peeled, cut into pieces, boiled 8 min	75	1 cup, 150g	21	16
	Tapioca, boiled	93	1 cup, 250g	18	17
	Tapioca, raw, dry	●	2 tbsp	25	●
	Tapioca, pudding, creamed, homemade	81	1 cup	35	28

★ little or no carbs   ■ high in saturated fat   ● untested/unknown   **G** GI Symbol partner

GISP	FOOD	GI	SAMPLE SERVING	AVAILABLE CARB (G) PER SERVE	GL PER SERVE
GREEN/SALAD VEGETABLES – LOW GI (LESS THAN OR EQUAL TO 55)					
	Alfalfa sprouts	★	6g	0	•
	Artichokes, globe, fresh or canned in brine	★	80g	0	•
	Artichoke, Jerusalem	•	3 medium, 145g	13	•
	Asparagus	★	100g	0	•
	Bean sprouts, raw	★	14g	0	•
	Bok choy	★	100g	0	•
	Broad beans, fresh, raw	•	½ cup, 55g	1	•
	Broccoli	★	60g	0	•
	Brussels sprouts	★	100g	0	•
	Cabbage	★	70g	0	•
	Capsicum	★	80g	0	•
	Cauliflower	★	60g	0	•
	Celery	★	40g	0	•
	Chillies, fresh or dried	★	20g	0	•
	Chives, fresh	★	4g	0	•
	Cucumber	★	45g	0	•
	Eggplant	★	100g	0	•
	Endive	★	30g	0	•
	Fennel	★	90g	0	•
	Garlic	★	5g	0	•
	Ginger	★	10g	0	•
	Herbs, fresh or dried	★	2g	0	•
	Leeks	★	80g	0	•
	Lettuce	★	50g	0	•
	Mushrooms	★	35g	0	•
	Okra	★	80g	0	•
	Onions, raw, peeled	★	30g	0	•
	Onions, stir-fried without extra oil	•	100g	0	•
	Radishes	★	15g	0	•

★ little or no carbs   ■ high in saturated fat   ● untested/unknown   Ⓖ GI Symbol partner

GISP	FOOD	GI	SAMPLE SERVING	AVAILABLE CARB (G) PER SERVE	GL PER SERVE
	Rocket	★	30g	0	•
	Shallots	★	10g	0	•
	Silverbeet	★	35g	0	•
	Snowpea sprouts	★	15g	0	•
	Spinach	★	75g	0	•
	Spring onions	★	15g	0	•
	Squash, yellow	★	70g	0	•
	Tomato	★	150g	0	•
	Turnip	★	120g	0	•
	Watercress	★	8g	0	•
	Zucchini	★	100g	0	•
GREEN/SALAD VEGETABLES – HIGHER GI (MORE THAN 55 OR UNKNOWN)					
	Broad beans, frozen, reheated	63	½ cup, 75g	1	•

★ little or no carbs ■ high in saturated fat ● untested/unknown Ⓖ GI Symbol partner

Acknowledgements

The information on stages of change on pages 73–4 is copyright © 1992 by the American Psychological Association. Reprinted with permission.

A book like this doesn't come along without a great deal of outside help. We would particularly like to acknowledge and thank Fiona Atkinson and the dedicated GI testing team—Anna, Marian, Karola and Kai Lyn and all our cheerful and well-fed volunteers. We would also like to thank Professor Gareth Dwyer for his invaluable help with the database. Special thanks to Philippa Sandall for revising and updating the text. Everyone at Hachette Australia deserves a medal for professionalism, but we want to single out our editor, Jacquie Brown, who gave it everything she had, and Fiona Hazard and Helen Littleton, ever active and committed on our behalf, making the vital strategic decisions that have made the *Low GI Diet* series the success it is. Thanks also to Vanessa Radnidge and Anna Waddington for all their work. We picked the brain of Professor Ian Caterson to distill the most up-to-date knowledge on the causes and treatment of obesity. Likewise, Professor Garry Egger (Professor Trim!) gave us his expertise on the role of exercise in weight-loss management. We thank Associate Professor David Ludwig at Boston Children's Hospital for his wise counsel and research on the GI and obesity. We are grateful to all the subjects who took part in our weight-loss trials—their efforts have strengthened our story and provided objective evidence of the benefits of following a low-GI diet. We would also like to thank Isa Hopwood who 'road-tested' the Weight-loss Plan. A big thank you to all our readers, colleagues, acquaintances and clients for their inspiring feedback on how the GI has worked wonders for them. Thank you to Julie Howard for the fabulous photos. And finally, thank you to all our 'success' stories.

And of course we wouldn't have made it through so many late nights and working weekends without the loving support of our families: a big hug and thank you.

Index

Recipe index